T0283844

PRAISE FOR *FRACTURED*

"Susan Mockler is a force—in writing, in life, in the world. *Fractured* is an unflinching look at the realities, both systemic and individual, of disability, and a testament both to the power of human will and to our need, as a society, to do better. Grace, determination, and power illuminate every page of this beautiful book. These words will stay with you forever."

—AMANDA LEDUC, author of *Disfigured: On Fairy Tales, Disability, and Making Space*, and *The Centaur's Wife*

"Susan Mockler's memoir is equal parts devastating and empowering. As she details her experience of recovery after a serious car accident, she fulfills a key aim of disability narratives by suggesting different paths forward. 'Recovery,' as she writes, is not 'a return to self,' but a reformation, a recombination of the shattered pieces to create an exhilarating, new whole. That's precisely what she's achieved here."

—ADAM POTTLE, author of *Voice: On Writing with Deafness*

FRAC TURED

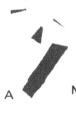

A MEMOIR

SUSAN MOCKLER

Second Story Press

Library and Archives Canada Cataloguing in Publication

Title: Fractured : a memoir / Susan Mockler.
Names: Mockler, Susan, author.
Identifiers: Canadiana (print) 20220203970 | Canadiana (ebook) 20220204055 | ISBN
9781772602708 (softcover) | ISBN 9781772602715 (EPUB)
Subjects: LCSH: Mockler, Susan. | LCSH: Mockler, Susan—Health. | LCSH: Spinal cord—
    Wounds and injuries—Patients—Canada—Biography. | LCSH: Spinal cord—Wounds and
    injuries—Patients—Rehabilitation. | LCSH: People with disabilities—Canada—Biography.
    | LCSH: People with disabilities—Rehabilitation. | LCSH: Spinal cord—Wounds and
    injuries—Patients—Psychology. | LCSH: People with disabilities—Psychology. | LCSH:
    Psychologists—Canada—Biography. | LCGFT: Autobiographies.
Classification: LCC RD594.3 .M63 2022 | DDC 362.4092—dc23

Copyright © 2022 by Susan Mockler
Cover by Natalie Olsen
Cover image copyright korkeng / Shutterstock.com
Editor: Diane Young
Printed and bound in Canada

The following versions of material from this book were previously published.
"Collision," *Ars Medica*. Toronto, ON, Spring, 2007, 94–101.
"Fractured," *Descant*. Toronto, ON, Summer, 2010, 149, 100–105.
"Hey Sexy," *Geist*. Vancouver, BC, Summer, 2015, 97, 14–16.
"You Oughta Know," *Wordgathering*. December, 12(4), 2018.
"Walking Class," *Disabled Voices!* Rebel Mountain Press: British Columbia, 2020.
A version of "On Disability" originally appeared in *Voices From the FOLD: A Festival Magazine*,
May 2021 and *THIS Magazine*, Toronto, ON, May/June, 2018, Vol. 51, No. 6, 12–13.

*Second Story Press gratefully acknowledges the support of the Ontario Arts Council and the Canada
Council for the Arts for our publishing program. We acknowledge the financial support of the
Government of Canada through the Canada Book Fund.*

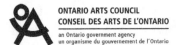

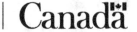

Published by
Second Story Press
20 Maud Street, Suite 401
Toronto, Ontario, Canada
M5V 2M5
www.secondstorypress.ca

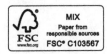

O body swayed to music, O brightening glance,
How can we know the dancer from the dance?

—W.B. YEATS
"Among School Children"

After such knowledge, what forgiveness?

—T.S. ELIOT
"Gerontion"

FRACTURED

AUGUST 20, 1995

WE DECIDED TO leave early. There was something about the sticky summer heat of the city, the restlessness I felt sitting on Gary's mother's couch, sipping decaffeinated tea, gray with milk, listening to Andy Rooney sign off on *60 Minutes*, that made me want to flee.

"Let's go tonight," I said as we drove back to Gary's. "Why wait until tomorrow morning?"

"Sure." He shrugged. "Maybe we can get to Vermont by midnight. Stay over and be in North Conway tomorrow afternoon." He reached around the gearshift and squeezed my thigh. "I like it when you're spontaneous."

His touch just below my cut-offs felt clammy, but I left his hand there and smiled. Impatient now for the cool mountain air, the stars silver against the clear night sky, I wanted this vacation. I needed this two-week escape from Ottawa, from my government job, and from the hollowness I'd felt since separating from Daniel almost two years ago.

Back at Gary's, I lugged a cooler to the car. "I grabbed a bottle of Chardonnay. And some cheese and crackers for when we stop tonight."

1

Surprise flitted across his face. "That's romantic."

By nine o'clock, we were on the road, Eric Clapton singing "Tears in Heaven" on a portable tape player in the back seat. The stereo in Gary's ten-year-old compact car had stopped working the week before, so I'd bought batteries, made tapes, and borrowed books on cassettes from the library. It was a long drive to the White Mountains. Eric Clapton was a compromise between our ages and musical tastes. I'd left some of Gary's favorites on his bookcase; I couldn't stand listening to "Hotel California" one more time.

"Do you want to stop for a coffee?" I asked after about an hour. "There's a rest stop up ahead."

"Let's wait until we're past Montreal."

"You're not tired?"

"I'm fine."

"I'll see if I can find somewhere for us to stay tonight." From the glove compartment, I pulled out a New England travel guide that I'd picked up a few days before. "Where do you think we'll end up?"

"Hopefully around Saint Johnsbury. But you might want to check on the Quebec side. In case we want to stop sooner."

I thumbed to the index, searching listings for Vermont. There was little light in the car, and I squinted to discern the names of hotels and motels near the border.

And then sometime between struggling in the dimness to read, sometime in that span of time between feeling the thin paper between my fingers, the smooth vinyl of the seat against my bare legs, the effortless turning of pages, sometime in that space from conscious thought and action to my next memory, the car hit a moose.

■ ■ ■

From a distance, someone was calling my name. I wanted to reply, to rise to the surface to greet the voice. But there was resistance as if a magnetic force were drawing me deeper and deeper into darkness: a darkness safe, calm, and unending. How easy to let go, to simply slip away, but I struggled and one thought formed: Not ready to die.

"Susan!"

I opened my eyes and returned to the world, trying to make sense of the chaos. Shouting, car doors slamming, flashing lights: red, blue, and bright white. The shape of a man hovering over me. Terrible. Something terrible has happened. I couldn't feel anything. I couldn't move. I was only mind. My body had disappeared.

Next, on an examining table, I gagged on something being forced down my throat. "Susan. Swallow," a woman said. "We have to insert this tube into your stomach."

Seconds? Minutes? Hours later? "Can we cut your clothes?"

Cut my clothes?

"Yes." My first word, raspy and faint. My throat raw from where the tube had scraped it. Then through the static of machines, the hum of voices, came the soft swish of shears.

"You're going to be okay. I know you're going to be okay," Gary said from somewhere nearby. "They're still trying to figure out what's wrong. You may just be in shock."

I moved my eyes to locate him. There he was, off to one side, only a few feet away. I'd forgotten about him completely. All that seemed to exist was the flurry of action between my body and the doctors and nurses.

I knew I could die. Any second now, I could be gone. But I wanted to live. I *really* wanted to live. "Please save me."

"You're doing great, Susan." It was the woman's voice again. My life depended on the skill of these strangers whose shapes and movements I couldn't bring into focus. "You're very brave. Hang in there. You're a brave girl."

Brave.

"We need to get her to X-ray."

The ceiling tiles flashed by as they rushed me down the corridor. Just like an accident victim on TV.

■ ■ ■

"Your right lung is collapsed. But you can live with one lung. No problem."

One lung. No problem. This murky new reality suspended between life and death, laid out on a table in an emergency room. This was me.

"We're sending you to the hospital in Ottawa by ambulance." The woman again. She must be the doctor, the one in charge. "They've called in the neurosurgeon. He should be there by the time you arrive. You'll be in good hands."

By ambulance? Back on the highway where this happened? Weren't there airlifts? But I didn't protest. Other people were making decisions for me now.

They packaged me up to be transported, to haul me back to Ottawa like a carcass; a slab of meat. As they loaded me into the ambulance, I overheard Gary arguing with one of the paramedics. They were refusing to let him accompany me.

"How am I supposed to get home?" Gary shouted.

"You're going to have to find your own way back, sir." The paramedic banged the rear doors and shut me in.

■ ■ ■

"He said he'd be here by three. His resident called him about an hour ago."

A different voice. I was somewhere else. Ottawa. I must be in Ottawa now. The room was diffusely lit. Two, no, three figures bustled around. I struggled to interpret shards of conversation. "Steroid drip.... O2 levels.... BP.... Catheter...." Impossible to assemble meaning from these fragments.

"He's here now. Call the porter."

"Susan?" A murmur in my ear.

"Mmm." Too much effort to speak.

"They're taking you down for an MRI."

Another room, this one flooded by light. The flash of a white lab coat beside me.

"Susan." A man's voice, authoritative and calm. "I'm Dr. Chamberlain. You're going to have an MRI now. Just close your eyes in there. That way it'll be over in no time."

They shifted me onto a table. I squeezed my eyes tight, then heard a mechanical *whirr*. And suddenly, somehow, I knew what they were assessing, what they thought was wrong.

"Susan? Susan?"

I blinked my eyes open. I was back on the stretcher.

"Susan? Do you hear me?" the doctor spoke.

Alert. I needed to stay alert. This was important. "Yes," I whispered. My breath was weak.

"There's good news," he said.

Good news?

"The injury is incomplete. The spinal cord isn't severed. And we don't have to operate. The fractures have decompressed."

Not severed. No operation. Good news. Incredibly, there was good news.

AUGUST 21

"I'M GOING TO WASH your hair. It's full of glass." A nurse spoke in my ear.

Glass? Glass? Of course...glass.

"Cut it off."

"What?"

"The hair. Just cut it."

"You'll regret that."

"I won't." I wanted everything simplified.

"It's easy to wash. I'll use a basin."

Steps echoed away, then the rush of water from a tap. Dark. It was still dark in the room. The night was endless.

"Your face was just scratched a bit." She dragged a stool over and positioned herself at the head of the bed. "Amazing really. There's so much glass."

I sensed trickling warm water, an astringent scent, and the nurse's fingers softly massaging my scalp.

"You have some finger movement in your left hand," she said. "It's a good sign."

I formed a fist with my left hand. Had the fingers moved? I was a stranger to my own body.

"If your arm recovers, you'll be able to transfer by yourself. You may even be able to live independently."

What?

A metal clang. The basin? "Almost done," she said, gently blotting my hair dry with a towel.

"I think you have enough movement in your fingers to use a call bell," she said. She held up a large plastic pad in front of my eyes. "This one is highly sensitive and responds to very light pressure. There. I just placed it in your left hand."

She had?

"Now give it a try."

I concentrated and squeezed. Again I felt nothing, but a beep sounded and a light flashed above me.

"You can do it." She reset the buzzer. "Get some rest now."

"You're leaving?"

"I'll be close by."

"Don't go. *Please.* Don't go."

"It's okay, Susan."

"Am I safe?"

"You're safe. If you need me, ring, and I'll come right away."

■ ■ ■

I awoke to daylight. The curtains around my bed parted, and two heads appeared.

"I'm Dr. Chamberlain. From last night? And this is Dr. Murray, my neurosurgery resident. Can you tell me your name?"

"Susan Mockler." Each word was an effort. My breathing was forced, my throat dry and sore.

"And where are we, Susan?"

"A hospital. In Ottawa." Ontario. Canada. World. Solar System. Universe. The way I'd decorated my notebook covers with my back-to-school Laurentian pencil crayons, the double pack.

"What year is it?"

"1995."

"And how old are you?"

"Twenty-one."

Dr. Chamberlain glanced up from his clipboard. "How old are you?"

"I'm thirty-one." Why had I said twenty-one? "A joke," I pretended. "I'm thirty-one."

"Okay." He wrote something down.

He probably thought I'd lost it. I had to focus. Control the way images and ideas kept distracting me, drawing me away. Then a kick of fear. "Brain damage?"

"There's no indication of that, but you have a severe concussion. You might feel a little confused. And you do have a spinal cord injury."

"But no brain damage. You're sure?"

"Yes." Dr. Chamberlain nodded.

Such a relief to hear that. That was something. Something good.

"But your spinal injury is serious," he continued. "Quadriplegia. Your arms and legs are paralyzed. And you have no sensation below your neck. Do you understand that?"

"Yes." I knew that my mind and body had disconnected. I knew that my systems had shut down, all functions replaced by tubes and IVs. I understood that. I really did. But nothing seemed real. "Will I get better?"

"Your injury is incomplete. So it is possible you'll recover more motor and sensory function below the level of your injury. If it were a complete spinal cord injury, there would be no chance of recovery. But it's unlikely you'll walk again."

"What?"

"You probably won't walk again. You need to be prepared for that."

Never walk again? Impossible. "Motivation? Does motivation help?"

His blank expression softened. "Motivation helps."

That was something too. Again something good. But everything was so foggy. And I was tired, so tired. I stopped listening and retreated to an earlier time.

■ ■ ■

We were ten, maybe eleven years old, my best friend Cristina and I were just old enough to ride the bus downtown by ourselves for a Sunday matinee: *The Other Side of the Mountain*. Images from the movie came to me with such clarity it was as if I'd seen it only yesterday.

Jill, the pretty teenaged championship skier, a corkscrew curve in the mountain where she flew off and landed, a twisted heap of legs and arms, poles, skis, and goggles. Her neck was broken and she was permanently paralyzed from the shoulders down. But after the injury she continued on: squealing with laughter as her boyfriend pushed her, running down the halls, wheeling her out of the hospital and into the streets;

and later, as a teacher, she answered her students' questions as she wheeled with them along forest paths. She was beautiful and loved. She had a meaningful career. A life in a wheelchair. But *still* a life.

I drifted away, comforted by the sounds of the swish of skis on snow and the sight of a young girl against a deep blue sky, gliding down a mountain.

■ ■ ■

"Susan." Another voice. This one familiar. Known. Beyond the nurses. The doctors.

"Mom…. But how?"

"Your friend Gary called me."

Gary? She didn't know Gary. Then a vague recollection from the ER. Gary asking for my mother's phone number, but the digits I'd known my whole life were muddled, impossible to retrieve. My mother's name, the street where she lived were all I'd remembered. It had been enough.

"There was a direct flight from London. I got here as soon as I could."

"You *flew*?"

"Yes."

"You weren't scared?"

"It was fine."

"I have a spinal cord injury."

"I know." Her voice cracked and she coughed.

"But the doctors say it's not severed. It means I can get better."

"We'll do everything we can. Hope for the best. I love you."

I couldn't keep my eyes open. "I'm going to sleep."

■ ■ ■

When I awoke, my mother was sitting in a chair beside the bed.

"What time is it?"

"Around four in the afternoon."

"What day?"

"Monday."

"*Yesterday* was the accident?" How was that possible? This distortion, this elongation of time? As if with the paralysis of my body, everything was slowing down, becoming still.

She nodded. "I should call Daniel. Shouldn't I? He'd want to know."

"Yes." He'd find out about Gary. But what could I do? Everything about me was open. I'd lost my privacy.

"Kathryn will be here tomorrow."

"From Vancouver? But she just started school. She doesn't have to come. I'm okay now."

"Of course." Concern flashed in her eyes. "It would be nice to see her, though, wouldn't it?"

They still thought I might die. Weary from the effort of thinking, speaking, I shut my eyes again. I'd tell my mother later not to worry, that I wouldn't let myself die.

■ ■ ■

I woke to the clatter of a cart entering the room and the patter of footsteps approaching my bed. My mother, Dr. Chamberlain, and the resident, Dr. Murray, introduced themselves to each other. I hovered in and out of awareness. Everything seemed so distant, as if my body was here, but I, myself, was very far away.

"I have a few questions, if you don't mind?" My mother's voice was composed but strained by anxiety.

"Let's step into the hall," Dr. Chamberlain said. As they left the room, I overheard a few of his words: "…still in shock…doesn't fully comprehend…."

"Okay, Susan," Dr. Murray said, "in terms of the procedure…."

Procedure? What procedure? I needed to focus.

"When we drill the holes, it will be noisy. But we'll freeze the insertion points on your skull first, so it won't hurt."

What?

"Susan. Do you hear me? Do you understand?"

Holes? Skull? I had to form a question, find my voice. "You're going to drill holes in my skull?"

"To attach this." He held up a metal ring. "The halo. It circles your head like a crown. We fix it with pins that are screwed into your skull, two in your forehead, two in the back." He took a frame, consisting of four long metal rods, from the cart. "Then we attach this to the ring and to this plastic vest that you'll wear. We put a piece of sheepskin under the vest, like a liner, to protect your skin."

"But…why?"

"The halo and vest immobilize you, so you can't move your neck or your head. That way the fractures are stabilized and have time to heal."

"How long?"

"Usually about three months."

Three months. Three months to get better? Three months! I forced the thought away. There was only now, what was happening now. "Okay," I said, as if I were making a choice.

Dr. Chamberlain returned. "Her mother said she's allergic to wool. I sent for this." He waved a small, furry, beige rug in the air. "It's acrylic, not sheepskin."

I was so glad my mother was here. I would never have made the connection between sheepskin and wool. Would never have remembered the itchy, red welts left by sweaters scratching my skin. That this had been part of me, of who I was: a woman allergic to wool, less than twenty-four hours ago. And now this. The abrupt rupture, the shattering of vertebrae, the concussion that made it difficult to access this memory: that the skin that was once mine was allergic to wool.

"Ready?" Dr. Chamberlain asked.

"Yes." Hopefully, this was the first step in reuniting me with my body, in making me whole. One nurse elevated the head of the bed while two others supported my body.

Dr. Chamberlain leaned close, his hot breath stale with coffee. He marked my forehead with a felt pen then indicated to a nurse where to shave the back of my head.

"You might feel a slight pinch when we inject the anesthetic." Dr. Murray prepared the syringe.

"I'm not scared." But I was lightheaded and the room was closing in. Then the prick of the needle as it pierced the skin on my forehead. I closed my eyes, waiting, listening. The murmurs of doctors and nurses. The rattling of tools and instruments.

"Can you feel this?" Dr. Murray tapped my forehead.

No. But I was floating away.

"Susan? Do you feel this?"

He wanted a response. "No," I whispered.

"Good. We're going to begin. You might feel some pressure, but there won't be any pain."

The drone of the drill. Closer and closer, buzzing in my ear. Then grinding, the crunch of metal boring into bone. As if I were a carpentry project, a chunk of wood. But there was no pain. Amazingly, no pain.

■ ■ ■

A cage. I was trapped in a cage. I couldn't move. Black steel bars framed my face. Help! I opened my mouth to scream, but then….

Monitors beeped. Tubes snaked across my body. Arms and hands lay limp by my sides. My stomach clenched. I remembered what had happened, where I was.

The halo telescoped my vision. I could only see straight ahead. I moved my eyes. My mother sat beside my bed.

"Daniel's here to see you," she said, getting up. "I'll be back later."

Daniel leaned over me. The shape of his face, dirty-blond hair, red-rimmed blue eyes, blinking with tears. "I'm here."

"I'm glad. Do you know what happened?"

"Your mom told me." His voice broke and he sank back in the chair, crying quietly. "The strangest thing is…it's like I knew. I was playing tennis at about ten o'clock last night and I got a sudden sharp pain in my neck. It was terrible. I had to stop. It was the same time…." He inhaled a ragged breath and sobbed into his hands.

"It's okay. Don't worry." Somehow it was easier to be inside the injury. Not to see what was visible on the outside. I knew I was still here.

"You know I love you." He rubbed his eyes, steadied his voice. "I'll do whatever I can to help you through this."

"I know." In my peripheral vision I could see him running his hands through his hair. Hands that had first linked with mine over ten years ago. Student-poor at the University of Toronto, scraping together ninety-nine cents each to watch double-features at the repertory cinema on Bloor Street, enough for a slice of pizza afterward if we were lucky. Since then, there had been love, anger, and a separation. Now this.

"There you are." No! Not Gary.

A screech of a chair against the floor as Daniel rose and stood at the end of the bed. Gary remained a few steps back. Absolute silence.

How had they recognized each other? Then I remembered: an office Christmas party a few years ago. Daniel was still my husband, Gary my boss.

Secrets colliding. The two of them here together. And I was stuck, powerless, incapable of running away.

"How dare you come here?" Daniel's face flushed with fury. "This is all your fault."

"There's nothing I could have done. And she doesn't want you here. You've hurt her enough already."

"What the hell do you know about it?" Daniel made fists with his hands.

"Stop. Please. Just stop," I said, but they didn't hear me.

My mom peeked through the curtains. "Everything okay

in here?"

"Make them go."

"Okay," my mother said. "Time to leave. She needs her rest."

Relief, such relief to see them go.

"I'm so sorry, honey. I should have been here. I had no idea Gary was going to show up."

"It's not your fault. I'm okay." But my voice shook.

"I'll talk to them. Figure something out. Do you want both of them to come and visit you?"

"Yes. But not together ever again."

"Don't worry. I'll take care of it."

I closed my eyes. I had to trust that she would make everything okay.

AUGUST 23

THE UNFAMILIAR SENSATION of motion. I wasn't moving, though. My bed was. The nurse had unlocked the brakes and was rolling me across the room.

She pushed the bed against the wall and pressed a button that raised my upper body slightly. "Now you can look right outside. See all the pretty flowers there." She gestured to the ledge that ran along the wall of windows on the other side of the room. "They're all for you."

I blinked at the streaming sunlight, moved my eyes to absorb it: the explosion of color. Never had reds seemed redder; purples more purple; greens greener. Tulips, irises, roses, chrysanthemums, potted mums in a wicker basket. The glimpse of blue sky, the brown drapes, the yellow walls. Everything so vibrant, like I was seeing shape, color, form, and texture for the first time.

I was shocked when I noticed five other beds in the room, two of which were occupied. I'd had no idea. Dim days, black nights, barely distinguishable. In and out of consciousness, beeping monitors, doctors, nurses, a scraping chair next to the bed as my mother, my sister, Daniel, and Gary rotated visits.

Brief conversations, a few quiet words. Yet the whole time I'd been curtained off in this space filled with light, objects, and even other people. I felt alert this morning, ready to become part of a larger world.

"What day is it?"

"Wednesday."

Wednesday. Sunday night was the accident; my mother had come on Monday; Kathryn had arrived from Vancouver yesterday and was going to stay for a whole week. Now Wednesday. Today was Wednesday. "What time is it?"

"About seven-thirty."

"And where am I exactly? I mean, where in the hospital?"

The nurse smiled. "The neuro-observation unit. It's like intensive care for neurology patients."

A neurology patient. That's what I was now.

■ ■ ■

The hospital routines were becoming familiar. Every four hours, the nurses logrolled me, placing me on each side and then my back, to prevent pressure sores that could erupt from the unmoving weight of my body against the sheets. Often, I was barely conscious during the maneuver, so seeing which direction I was facing when I opened my eyes could sometimes be a surprise. I awoke to see my sister in the chair beside my bed. "Hey."

She looked up from a magazine. "How are you feeling?"

"Better today. What time is it?"

"Almost noon."

"Have you been here long?"

19

"Maybe an hour."

Her eyes were puffy and red. Other than Daniel, who'd wept the first time he'd seen me, everyone was trying be positive, to hide their concern. "What's wrong?"

Her eyes widened, her lips tightened to a smile. "Nothing. Why?"

"What is it? You can tell me."

"Dad's here. We kind of had a fight, but don't worry. It's not a big deal."

"Dad's here?"

"He came this morning, while you were sleeping. I went to see him at his hotel. He was going on about how devastated Linda was and I just couldn't take it. I had a screaming fit at him. It's fine, though."

"When's he coming over?"

"Later this afternoon. He drove, so he's going to rest a while."

"I haven't seen him in ages." The last time was about five years ago when he and Linda kicked me out of their house. I was supposed to stay with them for the month of May while I was between apartments, commuting from their place in Milton to my summer psychology internship in Toronto. Everything seemed fine. My long days as a commuter meant I was rarely in their presence, but then after about ten days, my dad announced at dinner that Linda wanted to start getting the house ready for their baby, which was due in August. "We thought it would be better if you could find somewhere else to stay," he'd said, wiping his mouth with a paper towel.

I had almost no money and nowhere to go. I rose from the table and called my friend Lisa who lived in a studio apartment in downtown Toronto. "They want me to leave. Can I stay with you?"

"Of course," she'd said.

I returned to the dining room, hands trembling. "Lisa said I could stay with her. Even though it means she has to share her bed with me."

"I think you'll be much happier with a friend." My dad bit into a meatball. "Glad this worked out best for everyone." Linda stared at her plate and didn't say a word.

After that, I limited our contact mostly to Christmas and birthday phone calls. My father didn't seem to notice, or if he did, didn't seem to care.

"Susan!"

"Sorry. What did you say?"

"Are you glad Dad came?"

"I guess." But I didn't really feel anything. About my father. About the accident. One of the nurses had said I needed a "good cry," but I didn't feel sad. I had fleeting moments of panic, like brief electric shocks. I'm completely paralyzed! But I shut them down quickly, so they were barely perceptible. I erected a wall. Disconnected, so I wouldn't be overcome. I'd done this before. I was good at it. I was numb. Stunned. As if this were all happening to someone else.

■ ■ ■

My favorite nurse tugged back the curtain around my bed. The one who'd washed my hair the first day. Name. What was her name?

Brenda. I remembered! "This is my sister, Kathryn."

"We've met a few times." Brenda smiled. "I was wondering if you'd like to sit up today?"

"Sit up? Really?"

"What do you think?"

"Sure. Can my sister stay?"

"Why don't you go to the waiting room, Kathryn, and we'll call you back when we've sat Susan up."

A few minutes later Brenda returned, pushing a steel stand consisting of a pole about five feet high with two metal arms suspended at the top. Another nurse followed with a reclining wheelchair.

"This is called a Hoyer." Brenda wheeled the stand beside my bed. "We're going to use it to put you in the chair."

"How?"

"We slip this sling underneath you, attach it to the stand, and then use the lift to transfer you to the chair."

"Are you sure it's safe?"

"Don't worry. I got the okay from Dr. Chamberlain."

"It won't hurt my neck?"

"The fractures are completely stabilized. That's what the halo is for. You want to give it a try?"

"Yes." Though, I was apprehensive. But sitting up, it was exciting—a first step.

"Nancy," Brenda called across the room. "Come give us a hand. We're going to get this young lady out of bed."

Brenda and Nancy attached the sling, then supported my legs and upper body as the other nurse cranked the hydraulic lift.

"Be careful!" I blurted as I rose in the air for a terrifying few seconds and then they deposited me in the chair. They bustled around, strapping me in with a belt across my chest and hips, placing my feet onto footrests. I watched as they manipulated the body parts—my body parts—with an eerie sense of disassociation. Me. They were moving me.

But it wasn't me, either. More like being trapped inside a mannequin, a Barbie doll, though the halo, the blue gown, and the IV were unlikely fashion accessories. Barbie wouldn't be the patient. She'd be one of the nurses: efficient, competent, and stylishly outfitted in a white mini-dress, high-heeled pumps, a starched white cap with red trim, and maybe a stethoscope.

"There." Brenda attached a clear acrylic tray to the wheelchair and set my arms on it one at a time. "You're all set. How do you feel?"

"A little woozy."

"That's because you haven't sat up for three days. Your blood pressure drops with the positional change. But your body will adjust over time. We're going to keep the chair reclined at forty-five degrees to start with. I'll send your sister in and we'll see if you can tolerate fifteen minutes. Just buzz if you need us to put you back down before then."

Kathryn returned to the room. "How did it go?"

"Fine." But perspiration slicked my forehead and my stomach churned. "Can you ask them for some ice water? I feel a bit sick."

"Should you lie back down?"

"I need to be able to sit up again. I'll be okay." When Kathryn went to get the water, I cast my eyes downward and caught sight of my right arm on the tray. Black. It was completely black. I'd glimpsed the arm before as the nurses rolled me or changed my gown, but this was the first time I'd seen how bruised it was. From the sleeve of my gown just above my elbow to the tips of my fingers. Black. Entirely black. I still couldn't remember anything about the accident, but I must have raised my right arm to shield myself, must have had some awareness of the imminent impact. My right arm. Lying there flaccid and bruised, its last voluntary movement one of protection, a heroic, though ultimately futile, act.

I shifted my eyes to my left hand, palm down, the fingers flush against the tray. I willed the fingers, the thumb, to contract inward and watched the slow, deliberate response as joint by joint they folded under, forming a loose fist. Excitement shuddered through me. For the past two days I'd had to trust the doctors and nurses when they'd said that the fingers on my left hand could move and that my left foot had wiggled, just a little. I couldn't feel anything. But now, right in front of me, I could see it. My fingers moved!

I let go and the fingers and thumb relaxed.

"You're smiling." Kathryn placed a large, red thermal cup with a long straw on the wheelchair tray.

"Watch this. Watch my left hand." I focused again on the fingers and thumb and they curled inward. I contracted and contracted, and this time the resulting fist was tighter.

"That's amazing."

"Let's see if I can open them." But the resistance I felt trying to straighten them was so forceful, it was as if I were trying to unfurl them in a vat of rapidly setting cement. I groaned. "I can't do it."

"You will. You're getting better. I've never seen them move that much before."

My stomach lurched. The nausea had returned. "Can I have some water?"

Kathryn placed the long straw in my mouth. "Is that okay?"

"Mmm." The cold water was a relief, but I was still queasy. "Read something to me?"

"Like what?"

"Something from your magazine. Distract me."

"There's an article about O.J."

She leafed through the pages and tucked a strand of hair behind her ear. Effortlessly.

Until just four days ago, I had moved that freely. How was it possible that I had lost everything so instantly, so unexpectedly? Robbed of my real life and now imprisoned in this body, this living corpse. Stop. I couldn't think like that. My recovery had started. My left hand could move and I was sitting up. I closed my eyes and shifted my focus to Kathryn's words: O.J., Nicole, Ron Goldman, Ford Bronco, trial, Johnnie Cochran. Just a few more minutes and I could go back to bed.

■ ■ ■

"Don't wake her up. I'll come back." My father's voice.

"Dad? Don't go." A squeak as he parted the curtains around my bed. The room was still lit by sunlight. "What time is it?"

"Around three. Your mother said this was a good time to come." He hovered at the foot of the bed, radiating tension.

"You can sit down beside me."

"Of course." He moved toward the chair. "Linda sent this

25

for you." He held up a basket of perfumed soaps and bath salts.

"Thanks." A strange gift. Was this what had upset Kathryn so much? But he was the only father I had. Despite everything, I was glad he was here.

"How are you, honey?" He hunched forward. "I hear you're being very brave."

"They sat me up in a wheelchair today. I lasted for fifteen minutes. Tomorrow I'll try for longer."

"That's terrific." He leaned back in the chair. "And you have the right attitude. Be positive. That's important."

"Where are you staying?"

"There's this motel here at the hospital, for family to stay in. Only thirty-nine bucks a night. Nice clean room, even a mini-fridge. I slipped in a few beer in to keep cold." He grinned. "I ran into the maid, and she said it was no problem. I bet a lot of other people do that too."

He drummed his fingers on the armrest. "I brought you something else." He fished a brown glass bottle with a yellowed label out of his jacket pocket. "It's probably bullshit, but Monday night I was down at the Legion telling a few of the guys about your accident. Then last night this tiny, old Irish lady came over to where I was sitting and handed me a little bottle. 'For your daughter,' she said. 'Holy water from Lourdes.' I never believed in this shit, even when I was a kid, but she gave it to me, so I thought what the hell?"

"Might as well try anything."

"I'll just put it over here?" He placed it on the nightstand. "I should probably let you rest now. I'll be back in the morning."

"Thanks for coming."

"Well…I love you."

. . .

In my peripheral vision I could see the holy water, the flowers, and the plants crowding the window ledge. My mom had said that cards and telephone calls were pouring in. The visits were touching but unnerving too. Today, I had seen my mother, my sister, Daniel, Gary, and now even my father with his startling "I love you." He'd never told me that before. Tomorrow, Lisa was coming and other friends from Toronto next week. It was almost as if I were attending my own funeral.

AUGUST 24

EARLY IN THE MORNING, two doctors appeared at the foot of my bed. "Remember us? I'm Dr. Davis and this is Dr. Benson. We're from the rehab center."

I struggled to place them. So many doctors and residents showed up at my beside that they melded together, but these two were familiar, friendlier than the others. Both tall. Dr. Davis had curly, black, gray-flecked hair and bright blue eyes. Dr. Benson was blond and spoke with a lyrical accent. British, or maybe Australian.

"You're doing very well," Dr. Davis said. "Medically stable enough that we can place you in rehab very soon. You remember the research project we told you about?"

"Sorry?"

"If you agree, you're going to be our first participant in a study to promote walking in incomplete spinal cord injuries."

"Walking?" How could I have forgotten this?

"We'll suspend you in a harness over a treadmill. It's called a body-weight support system. We reduce the weight on your legs and then run the treadmill at a low speed while physiotherapists move your feet through a gait pattern. You'll get a better sense of it when you see the setup. How does that sound?"

"Incredible. When will it start?" A thrill fluttered through me. These doctors, unlike the neurologists, thought I might actually walk again.

"We'll admit you the week after next. It's an easy move. The rehab center is attached to the hospital."

"Great." Rehabilitation. Something to look forward to. Somewhere there was hope.

"I'd like to do a neuro exam with you now," Dr. Benson said. "We want to document any changes on a daily basis."

"I'll leave you to it," Dr. Davis said as he turned toward the door. "Bye for now, Susan."

I had only vaguely recognized these two doctors, though they'd obviously been here before, but the neurology exam was something I remembered clearly. Two, sometimes three times a day, doctors, residents, and medical students would encourage me to move limbs and test for sensation. This was a teaching hospital and I'd learned that I was an unusual case. A living, independently breathing, high-level quadriplegic. C1, C2, the two highest cervical vertebrae, were fractured. But Dr. Benson's need to examine me seemed less intrusive. He and Dr. Davis were going to help me.

"Let's start with your left side," Dr. Benson said. I watched as he placed his hand over the top of my foot. "Okay. Try to move it. The toes, the ankle. Whatever you can do."

I concentrated and tried to channel all energy, all will from my brain to my left foot. Move. Move. "Did it move?"

"Your toes wiggled and there's some flexion at your ankle.

Your foot moved upward a bit. It's better than when we were here yesterday. I feel very optimistic about this leg."

"I think my left hand might have improved too." I still couldn't feel anything but had noticed last night that it was easier for me to press the call button.

I tried to curl my fingers into a fist and open them again. Open and close. Open and close. I imagined the action in my mind and attempted to replicate the pattern.

"That's excellent," Dr. Benson said. "All the fingers are moving. Even the thumb. And you're getting both flexion and extension."

"So, my fingers opened? I couldn't do that yesterday."

"The extensors are still very weak, but it's a great start. Now, try to lift up your hand at the wrist."

"Did it work?"

"Not yet. We'll try again tomorrow."

"Oh." I wanted to be able to do that too. But today I had more movement than yesterday. At least on the left. Please let it continue. Please. Please let me get better.

Dr. Benson began testing sensation. "Tell me if it's sharp or dull?" He alternately pressed the dull and pointed edge of a pin against my skin, moving upward from my left foot.

"Nothing," I said. He continued along my left side. Not sharp. Not dull. I had no awareness of any touch at all until he reached a spot just below my clavicle. "Sharp. Sharp!"

"C3. The damage is below the level of the fractures. The MRI suggested that too."

He assessed my right side. Each touch brought a prickly, burning sensation.

"It's hypersensitivity due to the injury," Dr. Benson said.

"It should calm down over the next six weeks or so. It's a good sign. Tells us you've retained some sensation on the right."

"Why can I only feel on one side?"

"Your injury is consistent with Brown-Sequard Syndrome. For you that means your motor pathways are more affected on your right side and less on the left. Your sensory pathways are more affected on your left, less on the right. It's a rare condition, but it saved your life."

"How?"

"When the spinal cord is damaged above C4, the diaphragm collapses and many people die immediately. In your case, the diaphragm only collapsed on the right side, so you were able to take in sufficient oxygen until the paramedics arrived."

"And now I can breathe without an oxygen tube."

"But that's why the nurses keep testing your oxygen saturation levels with the clip on your finger. To make sure you really are ready to breathe on your own." He gathered his things. "We'll be back to check on you tomorrow."

Many people die immediately. My chest seized. I inhaled deeply, tried to relax. Breathe. Just breathe.

Their diaphragms collapse.

Just a few days ago, that had been me. I'd almost died. I'd really almost died. Dead. I could be dead. Gone. Consciousness lost. Not just my body. Nothing. I would be nothing at all. Just an absence in other people's lives.

My abdomen tightened as if I were encased in a steel corset. Breathe. Just breathe.

I *had* known. I really had known. Back in Emergency, I'd known that I could die. That right there could be the time and place where I ended. That each second of awareness could be my last.

But it hadn't seemed real. I was there, but not there. Disembodied, hovering above my body splayed on the examining table, above the doctors, the nurses. A nebulous fear, but mostly a blunted surprise at the incredible ordinariness of the moment. So sudden, so arbitrary, so unannounced. That this could be how it felt to die. So simple. So final.

Dr. Benson's words chilled me now. Penetrated with a clarity I hadn't experienced before. How narrowly, how randomly, I'd escaped death. How unlikely it was that I was still here.

■ ■ ■

Later in the afternoon, Brenda approached my bed. "I have someone who wants to meet you."

"Who?"

"Chris. Remember?" A few hours ago, she'd suggested I talk to someone who'd also had a high-level spinal cord injury to see how he was managing a year later.

"I told you I wasn't up to it." I didn't want any part of this, didn't want to have to make conversation with a stranger. But it was too late.

"Hi, I'm Chris." A sandy-haired man, maybe in his mid-twenties, with a light brown moustache and a lopsided grin, wheeled alongside my bed.

"I'm Susan." I moved my eyes to meet his. Chris used some sort of low-riding mobility device, part wheelchair, part scooter. A joystick rose from the center. A headrest supported his head and a urine bag bulged under his sweatpants.

"What happened to you?" he asked.

"Car accident. The car hit a moose."

"Whoa! Were you up north?"

"On the 417. About halfway to Montreal."

"Were you driving?"

"I was the passenger. But I don't remember anything. It's what I've been told. What about you?"

"I was driving off-road on an ATV. Not sure what happened, but I ended up in a ditch."

"Were you alone?"

"Yeah. I was in that ditch for ten hours before they found me. Can you believe it? *Man.* Ten hours, then they saved me." His eyes shone. "I'm doing real good now. Can drive myself around in this. And my left arm's pretty good too." With a jerky halting motion, Chris raised his arm from where it rested on the joystick. "My wrist goes up and down." He flexed then dropped his wrist.

"That's great." The action I'd been unable to perform this morning.

"Even ate a hot dog today. At the Rideau Centre. Held the bun and everything. I dropped it after I'd eaten about half, but my first hot dog. It felt good, you know. Got to keep trying new things."

I envisioned the basement of the Rideau Centre: the fluorescent gloom of the food court, the purple chairs attached to plastic tables, the neon signs of the fast-food kiosks. The high-school students lounging and smoking, the middle-aged shoppers sipping coffee, the mothers with strollers. All of them oblivious to Chris's triumph, where parked in a shadowy corner, he struggled bite by bite to eat a hot dog with his "good" arm. Ordinary life reduced to an almost insurmountable challenge.

"They treating you okay here?" he asked.

"The nurses are really nice."

"That's why I drop in when I come to the rehab center for an appointment."

"The rehab center? I'm going there soon."

"You'll get better there too. Just like me."

"I'm pretty tired now. I'd better rest. Thanks for talking to me."

"Good luck with everything. I'm sure I'll see you around." He backed up and pivoted to exit the room.

My throat ached and I tried to swallow hard, but my mouth was dry.

Chris had a story. He'd become what he'd survived. Now, like him, I had a story. Did it eclipse who I was before? Would it also define who I'd become?

What of rehabilitation and recovery? So focused on walking again, I'd completely forgotten about my arms. Arms were independence. Eating, washing, dressing. What if I could never do these things again by myself?

I needed to obliterate these thoughts. Closing my eyes, my mind reached out to my left hand. Move. Please move. There. I was sure that I detected the wiggling of fingers, stronger, more vigorous than even this morning. Who knew what would happen? How far this could go? Until time told otherwise, I had to hope for more.

AUGUST 26

"IT'S SUCH A beautiful afternoon. Would you like to go out for some fresh air?" Brenda held the long straw in the thermal cup up to my mouth so I could drink.

"Outside?"

"Yes. Outside."

"How?"

"Once you've built up your sitting tolerance, you can use a chair, but for now I'll take you out on a stretcher."

"I don't know."

"It will do you a world of good." She rang the nursing station. "Can I get a hand in here?"

A few minutes later, Brenda wheeled me out of the room.

"You're sure I won't slip off the stretcher?"

"You're perfectly safe." She and two other nurses had belted me in, tucked a sheet firmly around me, and raised the side rails. They'd elevated my torso to about a forty-five-degree angle so I could look around. But still, I kept imagining tumbling off the stretcher and crashing on the hard tile floor.

In the hall, antiseptic and bleach failed to mask the stench of urine and feces. Revolting. Did it smell like that in the neuro-observation unit? Had I just not noticed?

Brenda bumped me onto the elevator and both my legs shook. Panic choked me, but I pushed out the words. "What's happening?"

"You're okay, Susan. Just an involuntary muscle spasm at the sudden movement. It's part of having a spinal cord injury. Anything can trigger spasms and sometimes they happen spontaneously. You'll get used to them. Calm down and it will stop." She patted my right thigh.

We reached the main floor, and Brenda thrust me into the crush of the crowd.

Heads turned; people stared. I felt their eyes on me, heard their thoughts. What happened to her? I was a worst-case scenario. The metal halo-rods caged my face and protruded from my head like antlers. There's a person in here, I wanted to shout. Stop looking at me!

We continued on. Past the cafeteria, rattling dishes, clattering silverware, and more smells: grease and gravy, perfume and aftershave as others rushed past, dodged around me.

A final lurch and we were outdoors. I winced as the sun pierced my eyes. The breeze slapped my face.

"I want to go back inside."

"Give yourself time. It's a lot of stimulation. In a few minutes you'll be fine. We'll go over here."

Brenda parked me under the shade of a large maple tree and sat on an adjacent bench.

She'd positioned me well. Straight ahead between the bars of the halo, two black squirrels scampered across the wide expanse of lawn in front of the hospital. A white butterfly flitted among daisies, and purple coneflowers bloomed in a garden bed.

Then, my body jolted as the staccato roar of a helicopter ruptured the air. My legs quaked with involuntary spasms. At least now I understood how this new body reacted, what it might do.

Two boys, about six and eight, sprinted toward us to get a better view as the air ambulance maneuvered into sight and prepared to land on the hospital roof. But when they reached us, they halted, pointed at me, then at the chopper, their heads swiveling back and forth between the impressive machine hovering above and me, the monster with the jutting steel rods, just a few feet away.

I tried to smile, but instead tears wet my eyes. I blinked to stop them.

"I'd like to go in now." My voice was hoarse.

"Of course," Brenda said. "What a terrible racket."

■ ■ ■

Back in neuro-obs—in the fetid air, the dim light, among the beeping monitors and the other patients motionless in their beds, back on the other side of normal—I was safe, no longer exposed to the shocked faces, the scrutiny.

Out there I had longed to be invisible. It was a familiar feeling; one I first remembered from when I was about four years old. During one of my father's fierce rages at my mother—both of them drunk and disappointed—terrified by his loud shouts and the thud of his fist slamming into the wall, I'd lunged under the coffee table only to discover

I'd outgrown this refuge, could no longer make myself small enough to curl under there and disappear. So, I'd scrabbled to my bedroom, shut the door, and dove under the sheets, but it wasn't the same. I missed the comfort of the wooden table-top and sturdy legs of the coffee table, shielding me from my father's anger, protecting me like a shell.

But even then, young as I was, my body had agency, was an instrument of my will. I could use it to escape, to find a better situation. I could make myself safe, use my body to hide. Now, it was nothing; a lump under a sheet, barely keeping me alive. What if it stayed like this? What would become of me?

A pressure arose from deep within, an edgy blackness of anguish, of dread, forcing upward, tensing my stomach, gathering in my throat to form a howl, a cry, a shriek seeking release. I fought against it, squelched it down. I had to disconnect. Numb myself.

Yesterday, I'd asked the neurologist, Dr. Chamberlain, if I'd be able to work again.

He'd looked up from my chart. "It depends on the kind of work you do."

"I'm a government researcher, but I'm also doing my PhD in psychology. To become a clinical psychologist."

"That sounds like something you could probably do. But don't worry about it now. First, you have to heal."

But I did worry about it. I needed some kind of a life to aspire to, to visualize myself in, once I got through this. After we had spoken, I imagined myself in a wheelchair, or even with a cane and a limp, ushering clients into my office, maybe those who, like me, had suffered some kind of injury, whom I could help make well.

But after the outing today, this seemed preposterous. I was haunted by the eyes that had bored into me, their discomfort and pity; haunted by the shame of existing, a mangled body on a stretcher; worthless. Today, I didn't want to be part of the world. Today, I just wanted to hide.

AUGUST 28

SMELLS. I hated the smells. Of the nurses, the assistants, the aides. I choked on their perfume, their hairspray, was revolted by their sour breath, the nicotine on their fingers. I was forced to inhale the residue of their lives, compelled to submit to the intimacy of their care. I hadn't noticed it so much in the neuro-observation unit, but there had been fewer nurses, and I'd been less aware of my surroundings.

But now I was stuck for a week on the general neurology ward until I could be admitted to the rehab center. It had only been a few hours since they'd moved me here early this morning, but unlike the neuro-obs unit, with their quiet, gentle care, the ward nurses scurried in and out, an endless succession of strangers who didn't bother to address me by name. It felt as if they were warehousing my body, the remnants of me.

A young nurse bustled into the room and flipped on the light switch. "Wakey! Wakey! Time to wake up from your nap." She pulled on latex gloves and opened a catheter kit.

I was used to the procedure by now. They did it every four hours. A few days ago, I'd actually felt a sharp pinch while one of the nurses was inserting the catheter. Dr. Chamberlain had said it was a good sign, that sensation might be preceding function.

"*Ow.*" This time it really hurt.

"I can't quite grab it. Darn! I dropped the catheter. I'll have to get another kit."

She stomped out of the room leaving my legs splayed open on the bed. My cheeks flamed.

"I brought two more kits just in case," she said when she returned a minute later. She tugged on a second pair of gloves and again clumsily attempted to insert the catheter.

"You're really hurting me."

"You have a very small urethra. It makes it difficult."

"The other nurses could do it. Can't you get someone else?"

"Fine." She flung the second catheter to the floor and turned toward the door.

"Could you at least cover me?"

She tossed a sheet over my lower body with a frustrated grunt and stormed from the room.

A few minutes later an older nurse, maybe in her mid-forties, strode into the room, the younger nurse trailing behind her.

"I hear you've been giving Serena a hard time," the older nurse said.

"I don't think I'm the one causing the problem."

"I was just joking, dear. *Touchy.*" She rolled her eyes. Expertly, however, she inserted the catheter, drained my bladder, then measured and recorded the amount of expelled urine on a chart at the foot of the bed.

"What do we have here?" She pointed to a sheet of paper

taped to the whiteboard on the wall.

"Questions I have for the doctors when they come in on rounds. My mom wrote them out for me so I wouldn't forget what to ask."

The older nurse snorted. "How's that for patient empowerment?" She scanned my list. "What's this about walking?"

"I'm going to be in a research project at the rehab center."

"For walking? With your injury?" The nurse shook her head. "Last year we had a girl like you. Optimistic. Positive attitude. Couldn't face facts. And *she* never walked again."

Get out! I wanted to scream. But a stray hair brushed against my face, a slight tickle irritating the skin, forcing me to ask, "Before you go, could you rub a tissue against my left cheek? There's a hair or something there." My lower lip quivered, and I clamped my mouth shut. I wouldn't cry.

"Of course, dear," the nurse said. "Serena, will you get that? I'm on break now."

■ ■ ■

"You found me," I said as Dana, a hospital physiotherapist who had been working with me in neuro-obs, approached my bed. She was in her late forties with wavy, short blond hair and a voice that soothed me.

"Brenda told me they'd transferred you to the ward. I'll keep seeing you here. Until they send you to the rehab center next week."

"Good." Physiotherapy was the highlight of my day. Constructive, forward-looking, Dana was helping to prepare my body for what it would hopefully do next.

"We'll start with range of motion," she said. She stretched my arms and legs, fingers and toes, rotated my ankles, and flexed my wrists. "Okay, let's see what you can do. Start with your left foot." I tried to find a pathway, to send clear commands, waves of motion from my brain to my left foot, to my left leg. But without my limb in sight, I had no sense of the impact. Like screaming into a black hole, I received no feedback. I could hear no echo.

"How did I do?"

"That's good. Better than yesterday. Your ankle flexion has more range, all your toes are moving, and your whole leg shifted a couple of inches. Try the right."

I attempted to repeat my foot and leg actions from the left side.

Dana shook her head. "Nothing yet. But it's still early days."

"I know." The doctors had explained that recovery, if it happened, would take place in stages. Spinal shock occurred right after the injury. The area around the cord was bruised and swollen and no messages could pass below the level of the injury. Over the next six weeks, there could be a period of spontaneous recovery as the spinal shock diminished. More changes were possible in the first six months and then up until one or two years after my injury. Following that, any remaining losses were more or less permanent.

For now, time was in my favor; a promise of hope, but also of torment. I didn't want to wait for an unknown outcome. I wanted everything back. I wanted it all. My whole body back. Right here. Right now.

Dana lifted my right arm and held it steady. "Okay. Try

now." I focused, summoned energy, searched for a channel. Move. Move.

She shook her head and released the arm, setting it on the bed beside me. "Now for the other arm." She raised my left arm and positioned it in front of me so I could see it. She placed her hand in mine. "Squeeze as hard as you can." I curled my fingers around her hand and contracted them into a fist with all my might.

"Now open your hand." Extension was more difficult, but day by day it was improving. As I willed it in my head, the fingers slowly unfolded.

"How was that? Is it stronger?"

"The movement is smoother, less halting, but your grip is still very weak."

She held my forearm, just above the wrist. "Try to raise your hand up and back."

Wrist flexion. I closed my eyes and drew the movement in my mind. Opened my eyes and tried to execute it. Go. Go. My hand and wrist shuddered.

"It moved. I moved it. It wasn't just a spasm." A whisper of movement, but I'd done it. I knew I'd done it myself.

"No, it wasn't just a spasm," Dana said. "I felt the contraction." She grasped my upper arm. "Now, bend your elbow." Again, I closed my eyes. Move. Move.

"There's a flicker," she said. "Try again. Yes.... That's it. I definitely felt a flicker in your left biceps."

An anxious excitement rushed through me. The wrist and now this flicker. Neither of these things had happened before.

"Will…? Do you think…that…maybe the whole arm might get better?"

"Something's going on. Hopefully, something to build on."

Please let it happen. Please let me get back even just one arm.

■ ■ ■

"I called to arrange the TV service," my mom said, drawing the curtain back from my bed and settling on the chair beside me. "I paid for the week. After that you'll be in rehab."

"Thanks."

"They said it should be working in about five minutes." She checked her watch. "It's about quarter after seven. You could watch *Jeopardy* at seven-thirty, if you like."

"That would be great." I smiled. Watching TV like anyone else would be a welcome distraction. A return to the familiar.

"Do you want me to stay and watch it with you?"

"No, you can go. I'm so tired. I'll probably fall asleep right after."

"I'll get it set up." She tugged the arm of the tiny television that hung from the ceiling less than a foot above my bed and positioned the screen to face me.

"Do you need anything else before I go?"

"Just make sure the call bell is in my hand."

"It is," she said, glancing over to my left side. She placed the earphones in my ears, tuned in the station, and adjusted the volume. "How's that?"

"Maybe turn it down just a little…. That's good."

"I'll see you in the morning," she said, patting my arm. "Sleep well."

I moved my eyes to the screen. A commercial, an Italian grandmother cradling ripe tomatoes in a basket under her arm extolled the authentic taste and flavor of a jar of spaghetti sauce. The volume was a little loud, but not too bad.

Then the notes of the theme song blared in my ears. "This is *Jeopardy!*" The announcer's voice grated. The red, white, and blue flashing lights bombarded me. My head throbbed. I squeezed my left hand to depress the call bell. "I need help. Right away."

I closed my eyes, but my legs spasmed as the intermittent buzzers of the contestants reverberated through me like I was a tuning fork, suddenly struck.

Finally, after a couple of minutes, a nurse entered my room.

"Take these earphones out of my ears. Please. This show is too loud."

She reached through the bars of my halo and popped them out.

"Can you turn off the TV too? And move it away?"

"Is that okay?" she said, folding the metal arm and nesting the TV in the corner to one side of my bed.

"Yes. Thanks."

"Anything else?"

Suddenly I was aware that my mouth was dry. "Maybe a sip of water."

The nurse retrieved the thermal cup from the night table and placed the long straw between my lips. I drank deeply.

She set down the water and headed to the door. "Just buzz if you need anything else."

I took a few deep breaths and tried to relax. The sensory stimulation from the show had been intolerable, like being trapped inside a pinball machine. Was it because of my spinal cord injury? My concussion?

But the worst thing was that there had been nothing I could do to stop it. In this stunning new reality, I could no longer simply extend my arm a few inches to manipulate the controls or turn off the TV. I just couldn't do it. Not now. Maybe never again.

I flitted my eyes over to the TV where it hung in the corner, the screen now blank and lifeless as my limbs. I studied the space between my bed and the little TV, the inches that I could no longer reach across, the gap between what I now was and what I had been.

AUGUST 30

"TIME FOR YOUR meds." I heard the clacking of a cart as a nurse drew up beside my bed. I had no idea what they were giving me. There were shots in the morning and various pills throughout the day crushed in jam, so I could swallow them more easily in the halo.

"I don't want any pain medicine tonight." I moved my eyes, attempting to establish eye contact with her.

"What?" She fiddled with the pills.

"Last night they gave me something. It made me feel strange. Like I was hallucinating."

She studied my chart. "It was acetaminophen with codeine. You need to have it. It's too early for you to be off pain meds."

"I'm not in that much pain. I don't want it."

"I'll have to talk to the doctor." She sighed. "If he says it's okay, you won't have to take it."

"I think it's a mistake," the nurse said, returning a few minutes later. "But the doctor told me it was up to you. It's still on your list if you change your mind. Do you need anything else?"

"No."

"I'll turn off the lights then. Time for sleep."

Quiet. Now everything was quiet. Four hours to myself before the nurses barged back in to roll and catheter me. So good to be alone. I was almost always in the presence of others.

Even though I relied on the visits from my mom, Daniel, and Gary during the long days on the ward and loved receiving the calls, letters, and cards from family and friends, there was still a distance, a separateness. I felt connected, but apart. Even the people I was closest to were merely a backdrop to this new life.

What was most real, most present, was this; the time I had alone with this numb and motionless body, thinking of ways to influence it, to try to re-forge a connection. Last night the painkillers had put me in a dreamlike haze, but I wanted to stay clear and focused. My mind was the only part of me that I could still rely on or control. My body was now gone.

My body. How often I'd despaired of it, not thin enough, not pretty enough, not good enough. I'd been clumsy and accident-prone as a child, but my dissatisfaction with my body came later when I was twelve, maybe thirteen years old. I felt a collapsing hollowness inside as I remembered.

One night, coming home from my father's, I'd tried to be silent as I unlocked the front door. Creeping down the hallway, I'd hoped my mother was already in bed or at least passed out on the couch. But when I entered the living room, there she was, slumped in her chair, a drink in hand, a cigarette smoldering in an overfilled ashtray.

"So, who drove you home?" she propped herself up in the chair.

"Um…Dad's girlfriend."

"What about your father? Too drunk?"

"He was tired." Staring at the floor, I shrugged off my coat and unzipped my winter boots.

"What did she feed you?"

"What?"

"What did *she* make you to eat?"

"Dinner. Just regular dinner."

"Is she a good cook?"

"Would you stop it?"

"I thought she was a *marvelous* cook. Wine and candlelit dinners for your father. And here I am, stuck with two children. How could I compete with *that*?" My mother collapsed back in her chair, exhaling smoke.

"I don't want to talk about this."

"So, you're on his side?"

"Just leave me alone." I crossed the room, but had to edge by her to reach my bedroom. I could feel her eyes fixated on me as I shuffled past.

"You know," she said as she straightened up, suddenly alert, "the other day when your friend was here. Anne? The tall, thin one?"

"Yeah?"

"Well, I was thinking even though she's so slim, you actually could have a better figure than her."

"What are you talking about?" I shielded myself, folding my arms across my body, inching away.

"If you lost five pounds, maybe a little more, you'd be fine. Just diet a little. No snacks, smaller meals. In a month easily, you'd be fine."

"Would you *just* leave me alone?"

I slammed the door to my bedroom. Hot, angry tears spilled down my cheeks. Fat? Did my mother think I was fat? I peeled off my sweater and jeans and examined myself in the mirror, something I'd avoided since my body had started to change. But my mother was right, my stomach was softer, rounder than I remembered, my arms and legs were carpeted by an extra layer of flesh. I was disgusting. Fat! I hated myself. What I had become.

I pinched the soft skin of my upper arm, pressing firmly until a small red welt appeared. There. I grabbed another fold between my fingers, squeezing even harder, and with each stab of burning pain, the shame of my mother's words, and even the unease I'd felt with my father and his girlfriend at dinner, faded away.

So maybe that was the beginning—of self-loathing, of self-harm, my fingernails later replaced by razor blades. Stupid. So stupid. But I wouldn't think about that now.

My body was gone. And all I wanted was to reinhabit it, to be able to move it, feel it, make it part of me again. If it returned, I would value, nurture, and protect it. There must be *something* I could do to bring it back.

I shut my eyes, focusing on the energy, the buzz of neurons firing in my brain. I visualized this force, glowing and bright, traveling from the top of my head, along the base of my skull, passing through the contusion on the cord by the first two vertebrae, along the length of my spinal column, along the nerves through my abdomen and back, from my shoulders to my fingers, my legs to my toes. Luminous warmth flowed through me. Maybe it *was* working. I repeated these images of reconnection, this corporal mantra, and lulled myself to sleep.

∎ ∎

Muttering voices. I opened my eyes. In the faint light of my bedside lamp, a nurse was preparing a catheter. A second nurse stood across from her, resting her hands on the bed rails. I tried to ignore them, hoping to remain in the fog of slumber.

"We logroll her after this and that's it?" the second nurse asked.

"That's it," the first nurse said, tearing open a kit.

"What happened to her?"

"Car accident, I think. Check the chart."

"It was a car accident," I said.

"She's awake now," the first nurse said. "I told you to be quiet."

"What happened?" The second nurse gawked at me.

"The car hit a moose."

"Jeez. Were you up north?"

"No. On the 417. Between Ottawa and Montreal."

"A moose. *Weird*. Were you wearing your seatbelt?"

"Of course." I hated recounting the details of the accident, but felt cornered, required to respond.

"What happened to the moose?"

"What?"

"Like, did it die?"

"I don't know."

"Wow." She turned to the first nurse. "It sure makes you realize how lucky you are."

"Get out." My throat and chest were so constricted, I could barely speak. "Do what you have to, then get out."

I was just like you. Less than two weeks ago, I was you. And you, you could be me. If only I'd thought quickly enough to say *that* to her before she and the other nurse left my room.

I wasn't going to put up with it. Tomorrow I'd complain about this nurse and the one from my first day on the ward who'd ridiculed my participation in the walking study, ridiculed my optimism, my hope. How could they all treat me like I was nothing? I'm still here, I wanted to scream. I'm still here.

Other nurses and residents had grilled me about the accident. Had I worn a seatbelt? Had the driver been drinking? Taking drugs? Had I? No. No. No. But they'd repeat the questions as if compelled to assign blame. The truth of the accident, my injury, seemed to disrupt the illusion that they could safeguard themselves from tragedy.

For me, it was different. I believed what I had been told. The accident had just happened. A random occurrence in an uncontrollable universe. Nothing more, nothing less. I couldn't fathom a deeper meaning or explanation. I had done nothing to deserve this.

Last year, I'd attended a conference on women's health where a representative from a disabled association had spoken about discrimination, citing the ongoing trial of a man charged with murdering his disabled twelve-year-old daughter. "If they don't convict him, if they agree it was a mercy killing," the woman had said, "then that will demonstrate clearly how society views us—as not fully human, not deserving of equal rights. But just remember, every one of you, being able-bodied is a *temporary* state."

At the time, I'd thought of my ninety-year-old grandmother, her increasing fragility. But I was young and fit and like the nurse who had just proclaimed her good fortune, I had never imagined that disability was something that could happen to me.

Just three weeks ago, in what was now a different life, I'd visited London for the weekend after my grandmother had been hospitalized for congestive heart failure. On the Sunday, the doctor had informed us that she was well enough to travel to my mom's for lunch. I'd borrowed a wheelchair from the nursing station to wheel her the two-and-a-half blocks to my mother's house. It was a bright, warm, windy day, and my grandma huddled under a blanket, tucking her head down like a robin using its wing to shelter from a storm. I was dressed in shorts and a T-shirt and hadn't even noticed the wind. My grandma's reaction had given me pause. This was how it was to be old and frail: a strong breeze was an affront. But I was healthy and robust, I still had time.

I had never thought I'd be next. That in less than a month I'd be in a hospital; in a wheelchair myself. Never would I have imagined how unexpectedly and arbitrarily, how suddenly, it had become my turn.

If I could change it, I would. But all I could do was hope. Hope that I'd get better; hope that after this I could recreate some sort of a life. I guarded that hope within me, at times, frangible, at times, resolute. But I knew that without it, I'd plunge into a cavernous darkness. That without it, I'd lose everything.

SEPTEMBER 1

"MAYBE WE SHOULD give her lactulose?" One of the two nurses hovering by my bed said to the other, her brow furrowed. "What do you think, Patsy?"

"It's worth a try, Steph." Patsy stared down at me and shook her head. "You know if you don't have a bowel movement soon, you could get a blocked bowel. And then you'd need surgery."

"Surgery?"

"Don't worry," Steph said. She gave Patsy an annoyed glance. "Lactulose is a potent laxative. And we'll give you an enema too, to get things moving right away."

"I don't want to have a blocked bowel."

"Of course not," Steph said. "We'll go get the lactulose and the enema. Be right back."

"I'm scared to have a blocked bowel. I'm scared to have surgery," I said to my mother when the nurses left.

"I think that Patsy was exaggerating," my mom said. "I wish she'd just kept her mouth shut."

"The other nurse is nicer. Will you talk to her later? Ask her how long it takes to get a blocked bowel? If it really might happen?" I knew from the doctors that constipation due to slowed peristalsis was a complication for people with spinal cord injuries. But a blocked bowel? Surgery? Nobody had mentioned that!

"Of course, I will. Don't worry."

A few minutes later, the nurses returned.

"Do you want me to stay?" my mother said.

"I'd rather be alone for this," I said.

"Come back in about half an hour," Steph said to my mom. "She should be done by then."

"Here you go." Steph put a long straw in a cup and placed the straw in my mouth. "I mixed the laxative with apple juice. Try to drink it right down. It doesn't taste great."

Even in the apple juice, the lactulose had a phlegmy, sticky, and sickly sweet quality as it slithered in my throat. I tried not to gag as I pushed it down. "Okay. I'm done."

Steph removed the straw from between my lips. She and Patsy logrolled me onto my left side and slipped an absorbent blue pad under my bum. "Have you had an enema before?" Steph asked.

"No."

"This is it." She held up a clear soft plastic bottle with a slim nozzle cap that was about four inches long. "You might feel some pressure when I insert it and as the liquid enters your bowels. I'm going to insert it now."

I didn't feel anything, but heard a squelching, squishy sound.

"We'll be back to check on you in a few minutes." Steph placed the call bell in my left hand. "Buzz if you need anything before that." She and Patsy headed out the door.

Please let this work. Some gas escaped, a low, hissing sound. Good. That was a start. Hopefully something was happening in the void below me; a rhythm of internal movement that would release me from the fear of bowel blockage, of surgery. More rumbles of gas punctured the air. A smell, a putrid odor rising from below. Had the feces started to come out? I could only guess. The connection between me and my flesh, blood, bones, organs—this shape of a body I could no longer sense—was tenuous, but I needed it to keep me alive.

More gas and a stronger smell. Pungent, vile. I retched at the stench. That must be it. It had to be. I depressed the call bell and waited for the nurses to arrive to clean me, to report on the bowel movement, the measure of success. I tried to disconnect, to push away the horror of this moment, lying paralyzed in my own shit. How was this possible? How could this be me?

■ ■ ■

The lights were out. The room was dim. All I wanted was to escape into sleep.

"Oh…. Oh…." So far, I'd been lucky and had a double room to myself, but just after lunch an elderly woman recovering from a spinal surgery had moved into the other bed. So now, through the curtained partition that separated us, there was this: "Oh…. Oh…."

Stop. I wished she would just stop. Her moaning made me edgy. I couldn't relax.

"Nurse," she whined over the intercom. "Nurse. I need some help in here. Please. Oh…."

"Goodness, Millie. What are you doing?" the nurse asked when she entered the room.

"I'm trying to get up. I have to use the toilet."

"You're all tangled in your sheets. You're supposed to call for help if you want to get up."

"The toilet. I have to get to the toilet. I don't want to wet myself."

The walker squeaked as the nurse escorted Millie to the bathroom. Earlier in the day, a physiotherapist had helped Millie from her bed, and she had taken several turns around the room, groaning with each shuffling step, her tiny hands gripping the sides of a steel walking frame. "I can't make it back to the bed. Oh.... It hurts," Millie said as she and the nurse exited the bathroom. "Oh...."

"You're fine. Just rest for a moment.... There.... Okay.... Just three more steps and you're there.... Good job."

Good job? I couldn't stand listening to Millie's protests. She could walk with assistance and pee on her own. She had no right to complain, had no idea how much worse things could be.

The nurse settled Millie in bed. "Can I get you anything else?"

"I'm a little peckish, dear. I'd love a cup of tea with milk and a few of those biscuits the girl got for me last night. Would that be too much trouble?"

Tea and cookies! Did she think this was a hotel?

"I'll see what I can do for you," the nurse said.

"Here you are," she said, returning to the room after a few minutes. I heard the wheels of the over-bed table as she positioned it, the gentle rattle as she set down the cup and plate.

"That's lovely, Nurse. Just lovely," Millie said. "You girls are too good to me."

After the nurse left, I tried to shut out Millie's contented murmurs as she enjoyed her snack. But I couldn't, her little noises kept breaking through. Such simple pleasures seemed out of place. I didn't want to hear it. It seemed impossible to imagine that a day would come when I too might desire something as frivolous as cookies and tea again.

SEPTEMBER 5

WITH THE CURTAINS PARTED, my body positioned so I lay on my left side on the bed, I watched the clouds. When I'd first opened my eyes, feathery streaks trailed high above. Now, maybe a half-hour later, white puffs floated, each one separate, self-contained, sharply defined against the cobalt sky. Fair weather cumulus. Such a relief to reach back to my Grade 7 science class and remember.

The doctors had assured me that I didn't have brain damage, but my thoughts often lacked clarity. Images blurred, fragments from before the accident were lost. Just shock, they said, but I worried.

Cirrus, stratus, a Mackerel Sky. My recall was effortless. Maybe I *had* retained this part of myself. Despite everything else, maybe my mind really was still me.

Another memory: my hand shooting straight up in the air as Mr. Harris showed a slide of a funnel cloud. When called upon, I'd explained a detail that the science teacher had overlooked. Tornadoes could never come at night. Grinning, Mr. Harris corrected me. "But," I'd stammered, "my mother said...."

Head down, I'd stabbed a stubby pink eraser with the sharp end of the compass from my geometry set, twisting and twisting it, until the titters of the class had faded.

That evening I'd waited until Kathryn was in bed, until the opening theme music from *The Waltons* drifted into my bedroom, then charged into the living room to confront my mother.

"Tornadoes can come at night!"

"What?"

"Tornadoes *can* come at night."

"Don't shout. You'll wake up your sister." My mother sipped her drink. "What are you talking about?"

"You told me tornadoes couldn't come at night. When Kathryn was a baby and I wanted you to put her in the basement because of the storm. But they can. They can come at night."

"Well, I didn't know that."

"You lied to me! You're lying to me now!"

"What if I did? It was just a white lie. You were probably upset. You were always a nervous little girl."

"You lied. You lied about us being safe."

"Parents do that sometimes. I don't see why you're making such a fuss about it now." She lit a cigarette. "Just sit down and watch this show with me. I need to unwind."

"I can't trust you. I can't trust you ever again."

"Trust?" she scoffed. "Don't talk to me about trust. The person you shouldn't trust is your father. He's the liar. He's the cheat. Running off with that *woman*."

"This isn't about him. Why do you have to make everything about him?"

"He ruined our lives."

"I'm glad he's gone. You fought all the time."

"It wasn't that bad."

"He used to whip beer bottles at you!"

"He did not!"

"There are stains all over the wallpaper in the kitchen."

"He always missed. On purpose. And he *never* hit you or your sister."

"He did so." Though he usually apologized after, saying sometimes he couldn't stop himself from losing control. "We're both scared of him. You're not supposed to be scared of your own father."

"I've had enough of this. Turn up the TV, would you?"

I stomped over to the television set and cranked the volume to full.

"Not *that* loud."

"Fine." I rotated the knob. "Happy now?"

"Thank you."

"I hate you," I hissed on my way to my bedroom. I slammed the door and flopped on my bed. Rolled on my back and counted the white square ceiling tiles. One, two, three…. My mother was so weak. Why couldn't she get over my father? She should be happy he'd left. Four, five, six…. I would never be like that. I'd be independent and strong. I'd never need anyone. Seven, eight, nine…. Not now. Not ever.

But somehow, I did. At nineteen, I'd let Daniel in. Fully, completely, I'd loved him; I'd trusted him. And then, my first night on my own after Daniel had moved out, I'd returned to an apartment emptied of half our belongings and my childhood resolve had resurfaced: You can't count on anyone. You are always alone.

What if I never recovered? Lost my self-sufficiency? It was all I'd ever had. The one thing I'd thought no one could take from me. But right here, right now, it was gone. Completely gone. If I never recovered, who would I be?

My legs shook beneath the covers. My chest muscles gripped, like chains of a turning winch. Breathing was difficult. But I knew the spasm would pass. I needed to empty myself of worry. I refocused my attention outside, to a lone cloud towering high in the sky, and took slow, deep breaths. My body needed calm, peace, to heal. It was one thing I could do.

■ ■ ■

A few minutes later, I heard shuffling steps. A pale, plump nurse in a smock and matching pants appeared. She peered down at me. "I'm Martha. Your primary care nurse. You must be my quad."

Her quad? The noun was definite and uncompromising. Not merely an adjective, a transitional state, but global and permanent. A statement that annihilated anything else I ever was or could be.

"I'm Susan," I mumbled. Then firmly, "My name is Susan."

Martha rubbed her wrists as she scanned the length of my body. I represented a lot of work. The halo and vest probably added to my height and weight. With the halo attached, I must be at least 150 pounds and over six feet long. A cumbersome burden. A dead weight.

"Do you have a problem with your wrists?"

"Carpal tunnel, but it's some better now."

When I had been transferred to the rehab center yesterday, the admissions clerk had advised me that a primary care nurse would be responsible for me during rehabilitation. Martha was at least fifty. I'd expected someone younger, fitter. Could Martha handle me?

"Did you order breakfast? I don't see a tray here."

"No."

"They should have brought you meal cards to fill out yesterday. But I'll get you something now. What would you like?"

"A carton of skim milk and a meal replacement drink. Vanilla, if they have it."

"You need more than that."

"I don't really have an appetite. I haven't had solid food yet. I'm afraid of choking…in the halo."

"We'll start you out with soft foods. We have to get your system working. When was your last bowel movement?"

"There was something last week, but that's been it."

Martha frowned. "We'll set you up with a bowel routine here. That will help."

"What's that?"

"We give you a bulk fiber supplement, stool softeners, lots of water, and digitally stimulate your rectum to try to get things moving. We do it with all the quads."

Digital stimulation? The catheters were bad enough. Now this? Somebody's finger up my bum? I didn't want someone's finger in my bum. I wanted to be better. I wanted this to be over. I wanted to go home.

"I'll be right back with your breakfast," Martha said.

"I've got oatmeal and prune juice," she said when she returned. She set down the tray. "And milk and a meal replacement drink, just in case. First, we have to sit you up." She pressed the intercom on the wall above the bed. "Can I get a hand in here?"

Another nurse appeared and they rolled me on my back, then raised the head of the bed. I tried not to gag when Martha scooped oatmeal into my mouth. "Water, please." She slipped the straw between my lips. I sipped some water, chewed, and swallowed. "I did it. I got it down."

"That's really good. We'll take it slow."

A mouthful of oatmeal, a sip of water. After a few minutes I cast my eyes down to the tray. "I've eaten almost half the bowl!"

Martha smiled and nodded, then picked up a moistened facecloth and dabbed the corners of my mouth and chin where I'd dribbled oatmeal.

Spoon-fed! I was being spoon-fed! "I've had enough." A glob of congealed oatmeal felt lodged in my throat. "Just some water, please."

"That's fine. You ate a good amount." She cleared the tray, lowered the head of the bed, and retrieved a basin from the cupboard. "I'm going to get everything ready for your bed bath."

I heard the gush of water as she filled the basin in the bathroom. I concentrated on squeezing my left hand into a fist, then releasing it and attempting to straighten my fingers. I tried to lift my hand up at the wrist. I couldn't see my hand or arm from where I lay. Had it worked? I had no idea. The torture of unknowing.

Please come back to me. Just one hand. Just one arm. Just on the left. Please come back. Please come back and I'll be okay.

Martha set the basin and a small pile of white washcloths and towels on the nightstand. She reached behind the halo to loosen the tie of my blue hospital gown, and slipped it off. She wet the washcloth and drew it over each of my eyelids. She rinsed and soaped the cloth and I felt warm, wet strokes as she washed my face, neck, and ears.

The nurses on the neurology ward had wiped me down daily, but Martha was different. Methodical, meticulous, yet gentle as she washed, rinsed, and towel-dried each body part in turn. In the same way she would bathe an infant. My right leg shook.

"A bit of a spasm," Martha said. "Don't worry. You're fine."

But I wasn't fine. Far from it. This was only temporary. It had to be.

As Martha plodded through her tasks, brushing my teeth, my hair, I felt a quiet sadness emanating from the soft creases in her face, her pallid blue-gray eyes, as if life had been a series of mundane disappointments, flat and tiring. A thin gold band cut into her fleshy fingers. What would I learn about Martha as the months passed? Although thrown together by necessity rather than choice, unlike the brief interactions with the staff on the ward, my relationship with Martha would be more enduring. She was someone that I would have to get to know.

"There was another Susan here, about the same age as you," Martha said as she tidied up. "She left yesterday."

"I think I saw her. Does she have a spinal cord injury too?"

"No. She has MS. She had a relapse. She's been in here a few times before. But it might have been nice for you to have another girl to talk to. Mostly, it's men here. Young men. They take risks, do reckless things, and end up here."

I didn't really mind that there were no other women here. I didn't care about making friends. I preferred to keep to myself. But I had noticed her, this other Susan. I was propped up on a stretcher, having been wheeled over here from the hospital. The porter had parked me in the hallway while the cleaners readied my room. A woman with shoulder-length black hair and thick, black-framed glasses had wheeled out of the room two doors down from mine. Her mother walked with her, dragging a large suitcase. A few minutes later, her father exited her room, his arms piled high with boxes of disposable adult diapers. In that moment, I had hoped that I wouldn't be discharged with diapers when it was my turn to leave here. But, of course, I knew that I might.

"Time for you to get dressed," Martha said. "How's this outfit?" She held up a pair of red, plaid, flannel boxer shorts and a white T-shirt she'd selected from the clothes my mother had brought in. The T-shirts had been altered with a slit to fit over the halo.

"Usually, they keep me in a hospital gown."

"Well, now you'll be getting dressed. Look, the T-shirt matches your TEDs." She pointed to my legs which were encased in white compression stockings. The stockings, along with blood thinners, would prevent the formation of blood clots in my legs. Although I was out of immediate danger from my injury, there were still many ways to die.

Martha wiggled running shoes onto my feet and tied the laces. "It's taken us almost two hours, not bad for the first day." Perspiration glistened on her upper lip and crescent-shaped stains dampened her underarms. "You're ready to go."

"Where?"

"You're due in physio at eleven." She checked her watch. "We just made it. I'll get you a chair. You've been using a reclining one?"

"Yes."

"They'll fit you with your own chair in OT this afternoon."

"OT?"

"Occupational therapy."

Occupational therapy? I didn't know much about it except for what I'd seen in the movies: patients weaving baskets, building birdhouses, or making crafts. Now, it was somewhere for *me* to go?

Martha and another nurse returned to the room.

"Where's the lift?" I asked.

"We don't use them. We'll do a two-person transfer with this." Martha indicated a rectangular piece of plywood, about ten inches wide and maybe two and a half feet long. "A sliding board."

"You're sure you can do this?"

"We've transferred quads twice the size of you," the other nurse said.

Martha wheeled the chair beside the bed, locked the brakes, and removed the armrest closest to me. My legs trembled slightly, unnerved by yet another unanticipated trial. But after spending the morning in her care, I now trusted Martha completely, despite her weakened wrists. Her presence comforted me. I knew she would keep me safe. She and the other nurse wedged the board under me to create a bridge, slid me across the board and into the chair, and belted me in at the waist and chest.

"See?" Martha smiled. "Piece of cake."

They had executed the transfer expertly, but I hated having to be handled this way, a lifeless lump of flesh. I was still here, still present. But where was I located? Did the outline of my body, the surface of my skin, contain me or did I exist only within what remained intact, the undamaged brain, the repository of mind?

Martha slid a clear acrylic tray over the armrests and placed my arms on it one at a time. "If they're not supported, the weight of your arms can dislocate your shoulders," she said.

I stared at my arms, my hands, these new threats. I closed the fingers of my left hand. Then opened them. Slowly, the fingers and then the thumb straightened. It was getting easier! I lifted my hand at the wrist. Like last week, there was a tremor. Something was happening there. I concentrated on the right, trying to coax some movement, but the hand lay flaccid on the tray, bloated and discolored like a dead fish.

"The porter should be here soon." Martha placed the call bell under my left hand. "Do you need anything else?"

"No. Wait. Is that a mirror on the closet door?"

She nodded.

"Can you wheel me in front of it? I haven't seen myself since…. Oh no…. But…no one told me." My face was distorted, puffy, and mottled purple, yellow, and green with red slashes of healing cuts across my forehead and the bridge of my nose.

"The swelling will go down," Martha said. "It takes time. That's all."

I searched the eyes gazing back at me from between the bars of the halo. Was there some flicker of familiarity? I'd expected to look different. I knew that my hair was no longer loose at my shoulders, but bound back in a ponytail to avoid strands tickling my skin. I wore glasses secured by an elastic cord, not contacts. And of course, there was the halo and the useless body strapped into a wheelchair. I knew all this. But my face? Why had no one warned me? I was barely recognizable. What else were they keeping from me?

"Do you want me to move you?" Martha asked.

"No." I studied the reflection to find some quality, some remnant, I could identify as myself.

SEPTEMBER 7

"SHOULD I MAKE us our peppermint tea?" my mom said, holding up the box with the striped candy cane on the front.

"Sure," I said.

Over the past couple of days, we'd developed a nightly routine. My dinner was delivered to my room around 5:30 and, spoonful by spoonful, my mom fed me. The vegetarian meals I requested were usually some combination of lentils, beans, and rice cooked to a flavorless mush. I didn't care. I only wanted food that was easy to swallow. My goal was to finish half my meal and drink a small carton of milk, hoping the calcium would help my fractured vertebrae heal. My mom put my long straw in the often-lukewarm milk and I sipped until I got it all down. After I'd finished with the ordeal of eating, we had tea.

"Here we are," my mom said, placing the thermal cup on the tray of my wheelchair. Steam rose from the opening and I inhaled the crisp scent of mint.

"I brought us a treat from the hospital cafeteria." She withdrew a large piece of plastic-wrapped chocolate cake with chocolate icing and two forks from her purse.

"I can't eat that," I said. "But go ahead. It looks great."

"Why don't you want it?"

"I'm allergic to chocolate."

"But you loved chocolate as a little girl."

"I'm allergic to it now."

"Since when?"

"I don't know. Since I was about seventeen."

"You never told me. I would have remembered."

"Maybe." But maybe not. She'd only been sober for five years. She'd forgotten a lot from before. Though, she had remembered my allergy to wool.

"If you'd told me, I would have gotten something else. Like carrot cake. Do you still eat that?"

"Don't worry about it. I just want tea. I still don't have much of an appetite."

She slipped the long straw into my cup.

"Be careful. It may be too hot."

"I know." I took a small sip. "It's fine."

"I'll just have tea too," she said, rewrapping the cake. "I'll eat this later."

After a few minutes, she fished some letters out of her purse. "You got a letter from Grandma today. Would you like me to read it?"

"Are there any from Margie?"

She shuffled through the letters. "There's one here."

"Start with that." Margie was my second cousin. I'd never met her and probably never would. But she wrote faithfully to her grandfather, my grandmother's older brother, and he forwarded the letters to my grandma who now sent them to me.

Margie was about my age and, like me, had recently separated from her husband and was rebuilding her life.

Dear Grandpa,

I'm glad to hear you are learning French. Not too many ninety-four-year-olds can say that!

Things are going well for me. I just moved to the first floor of a house near High Park. It's an old, renovated house and very nice. I've started running with a club and am training for a half-marathon. I'm doing 10k every morning!

My mom paused and looked over at me.

"That's probably enough for now," I said. "I'll call the nurses to get me ready for bed."

"I'll just pop out for a cigarette."

When my mom returned, Trish, one of the night nurses, was brushing my teeth with the electric toothbrush my mom had bought last week.

"I can do that," my mother said.

"That's okay. We're all finished here," Trish said. "Do you need anything else?"

"No. Thanks," I said.

After Trish left, my mom held up a plastic bottle. "Vitamin E capsules. I talked to the pharmacist today and she said that breaking these open and rubbing the liquid on your cuts would prevent scarring much better than Vitamin E cream. Should we try it?"

The last thing I worried about was whether my face would be scarred. But my mother was concerned, had mentioned it several times. And maybe she was right. Maybe someday I'd care about my appearance again.

She split a capsule in half and dabbed the liquid on my forehead between my eyebrows and along the left side of my nose. She squinted, examining me the way she had when I was a child, scanning for any residue of ice cream or ketchup. She'd pull a scraggly tissue from her purse, fusty with face powder and tobacco shreds, wet it with saliva, and wipe away any smears. How I'd hated that!

Even now I bristled a little at her touch. I didn't want to but couldn't help it.

I tried to focus on this mother who was devoted, steady, and reliable, the one I desperately needed and could count on. But I couldn't stop the memories of the mother from the past whose words and actions had marked me as indelibly as a tattoo. They had endured and become a touchstone of self: unloved, unwanted. I'd survived, become callused, indifferent. I'd disconnected from her, disconnected from my vulnerability, and my dependence. I'd become strong and free.

I wanted to forget, I wanted to forgive, but I couldn't eradicate her impact on me any more than I could make the mother from the past completely disappear.

■ ■ ■

"Where's the social worker?" I asked when my mother entered my room the next morning. "I thought she was coming at ten-thirty."

"My appointment with her ran a little over time. She'll be up in a few minutes."

"What's that?" I asked. My mom carried a large black binder.

"Just something she gave me. About living with quadriplegia." She slid it on a closet shelf. "I told her we didn't need it. That we'd see how well you recover, then go from there. It's too early now."

"That's why I don't want to meet with her yet. I don't really want to talk about anything until I know how I'll be."

My mom sank in a chair and closed her eyes.

"Are you tired?"

"A little."

"Did she say anything else?"

"Not really. Just that I should spend time taking care of myself—go to a movie, for a walk, shopping, something like that."

"Maybe you should? You don't have to always be here."

"I've been coming in later in the mornings. But as I told her, I want to be here. I don't want to be anywhere else."

I felt a pang of guilt.

Heels clattered in the hall. "I think she's coming now," I said.

"Good afternoon. I'm Connie Schwimmner." A middle-aged woman poked her canary-colored head into the room. "You must be Susan. Mind if I come in?"

"This is my mother…."

"I know. We became chums downstairs."

"You're here to do the power of attorney with us?"

"Righty-o. I'll set up over here." She arranged some

papers on my over-bed table and pulled over a chair. "This is how it works."

I half-listened as Connie detailed the nature of the transfer of power of attorney: one for health and one for finances. My mom had explained it to me already. In my case, this was a temporary arrangement, not related to my ability to make my own decisions, but simply so that my mother could sign forms and write checks for my rent and bills until I was out of the rehab center. Then I'd resume doing things for myself.

"...these documents are kept in a fire-proof cabinet in the records department. So, if you're in another accident or become incapacitated again in the future, they will always be here." Connie caught my eye and smiled.

"What?"

"I was just saying—"

"I know what you said. Let's focus on *this* accident for now."

"Of course, dear." Connie set the forms on the tray of the wheelchair. "Now, if you'll sign here."

Sign? "I can't." I stared at the forms in disbelief. "I can't."

"Can she make an *X*?" Connie turned to my mother.

"No," I said. "I can't."

My mom cupped my shoulder. "What if we put a pen in your hand and move the paper underneath. Would that work?"

"Sure." Connie said.

I curled my hand, and my mother wedged the pen between my fingers. I gripped it with all my strength. Hold. Hold. Hold.

Connie traced an *X* in the first signature space. "Just one more," she said, flipping the page.

My hand trembled. The pen started to slip. "Oh no!" I said. Hold. Hold. Please. Just hold.

My mother covered my hand with hers and steadied the pen. "Okay, Connie. Do the other one now."

Again, Connie traced an *X* in the space where my signature belonged. An *X*; anonymous, nameless. I had become merely an *X*.

Connie gathered the papers together. "I'll just witness these and be off," she said. "I'll send copies up later."

"Can you wheel me to the window?" I asked my mother.

My mom unlocked the brakes of my wheelchair and pushed me across the room.

"Is this where you want to be?" She angled the chair so I could peer out.

A few russet-edged maple leaves skittered across the lawn. Already? The trees were changing already? Summer was cycling into autumn without me. While I'd been imprisoned here. Motionless and still.

I didn't want to be here. I wanted to be away. Away from this room, this paralysis, away from Connie, the papers. Away from everything. But I was trapped. No chance for escape.

"Don't worry," my mom said. "You'll be signing your own name soon. We just have to be patient."

"I know," I said, going along with her. But I'd seen the shock in her eyes, mirroring my own, when Connie had requested my signature. "I think I'll lie down. Can you ask the nurses to come in and transfer me on your way out?"

"Sure, honey. I'll be back later."

The two diagonal lines, crossed at the center loomed in my mind. An *X*! I couldn't even make an *X*. My legs trembled.

So stupid. I was so stupid. My progress had given me too much hope. Stuck in rehab, I hadn't realized how incapable I was of functioning in the outside world. Useless. I was utterly useless. Without a signature, I was nothing.

And what if I didn't get any better? What if I had to return to my mother's home, helpless and as vulnerable as I'd been as a child?

I couldn't. No matter how hard my mother was trying to get it right this time, I just couldn't do it. I'd rather die.

SEPTEMBER 11

MARTHA HAD JUST removed my lunch tray and cleaned my face with a damp cloth, when Peter, a colleague from work, rapped at my half-opened door.

"Come in," I said, and he wheeled into my room.

Before the accident, Peter was the only person I knew well who used a wheelchair. A soft-spoken man in his late forties with a gentle sense of humor, I'd consulted with him on a number of research projects. I'd never really thought about his disability or the fact that he used a wheelchair. It was just part of who he was. Seeing him now though, I noticed details about him that I hadn't before I understood the critical distinctions: quadriplegia, paraplegia, complete, and incomplete. Peter had a manual chair, and though he used his arms, his hand movements were compromised, and two of the fingers on his left hand curled under in a spasm. He was an incomplete quad—like me.

"I brought you this." He held up a package of peppermint tea. "Should I leave it on the table here?"

"Thanks so much. My mom and I drink peppermint tea every night. It's like you knew."

He pulled up across from me and applied the brakes on his chair. "So how are you coping with all this?"

"Okay, I think. Just focusing on rehab. I'm getting some movement back on my left side."

"Ahh…rehab." His face crinkled with a smile. "The old heave-ho. I don't imagine things have changed much since my time."

"No." I didn't mention that soon I'd be doing body-weight support training, exploring the possibility of walking. It didn't seem fair.

"What level is your injury?" he asked.

"C1/C2. What's yours?"

"C6. You know, you're the first person I've known to have a spinal cord injury since my own accident…almost thirty years ago now."

"What happened?"

"I'd just turned nineteen—my first year at university in Vancouver and I was working ski patrol that winter. The slopes had closed for the day and a few of us were goofing around, showing off, doing jumps. It was very icy, and I crashed. That was it. We shouldn't have been doing it, but kids…. They think they're invincible."

"Were you in rehab long?"

"Four or five months. I went back to school the next fall. Life went on. And kept going on. And you know, Susan, I've been pretty happy. I have a good life."

I knew from our conversations that Peter was married, had a job he loved, drove a modified van, and traveled extensively for work and for holidays.

"And you will too," he said. "There's one thing that

another fellow told me after I was injured that I'll never forget. 'There are probably over a million things you can do in life. Maybe more. Now there may be a couple of thousand things you can't do, but you can still do everything else.'"

"That's a good way to look at it."

"It helped me a lot. Especially during my darker times. I hope it helps you too." He released the brakes on his chair. "I should let you get back to it. I'll come again."

"I'd really like that. And...thanks. Thanks for everything."

A skiing accident. Thirty years ago. C6 incomplete. Peter's vital statistics. Whenever I met someone else at the rehab center with a spinal cord injury, these were the first facts we exchanged. What happened? When? What level?

But in the years I'd known Peter, I'd never thought to ask him what had happened to him or why he used a wheelchair. In the outside world, at work, it didn't seem to matter. He'd moved beyond his story, beyond being defined by his injury. One day I hoped to be like that too. Just existing like everyone else, not having to explain.

∎ ∎ ∎

"That's the girl I told you about," I said to my mother as we waited for my afternoon physio appointment. On the other side of the room, a young paraplegic girl was working with her physiotherapist.

"Who is she again?"

"The one from up north who was up all night crying? Whose mother wasn't here with her?"

"Poor thing. Is her mom here now?"

"I'm not sure."

A few nights ago, when I'd been trying to sleep, the usual late-night silence had been shattered by wracking sobs from down the hall. Even though the door to my room was shut, the explosive crying had intruded. I couldn't plug my ears. I couldn't bury my head under the covers. I had no choice but to be bombarded by the relentless wailing. My body tensed. I needed my sleep. Be quiet. Please. Just be quiet.

I pressed the call bell. "Can I have some Gravol?" Gravol helped me to relax, to drift off to sleep.

"Be right there," Lucy, one of the regular night nurses, said through the intercom.

A few minutes later, she entered my room and started preparing the Gravol, crushing it so it was easy for me to swallow.

"Who's crying?" I asked.

"The new admission. Just came over from the hospital today. She's only sixteen. We're trying to do what we can for her, but she's scared. She wants her mother. It's heartbreaking."

"Where is her mother?"

"Well, she was here but had to go back up north for a few days. They live somewhere near Timmins. There are four other younger kids. She has to sort things out before she can come back again."

After Lucy left, I closed my eyes and tried once again to ignore the girl's sobs. Her weeping was softer now, more of a whimpering, not unlike that of a wounded puppy. I didn't want to hear her pain, her sounds of suffering. I wanted her to stop. She didn't know it yet, but she'd have to be stronger, tougher. She was just at the beginning. She had a long way to go.

When I'd seen her the next day in the corridor, hunched in a wheelchair, her eyes looked punched from crying; red, swollen, and half-shut. But today she was bright-eyed and giggled at something her physiotherapist had just said. I was surprised by the difficulty of her exercises: side-lying leg raises, hamstring curls. I'd done them myself, before, in aerobics classes. They weren't easy.

Then she sat on the edge of the bed and stood up! She actually stood up and began walking. I was stunned.

"Mom. Look! She's walking!"

"What? Wasn't she just admitted?"

"I guess her injury was minor. She probably came out of spinal shock."

She walked the length of the room then returned to join her physiotherapist. She wasn't even unsteady. She looked like any other teenage girl who was just walking.

My mother picked up a magazine and rifled through the pages. "She seems fine. Why haven't they discharged her yet?"

"Maybe she needs to build up her strength."

"Well, she could do that somewhere else. She shouldn't take up a space. Another person might really need it." My mother was unusually harsh, but I understood. This girl's speedy return to normal stung. Both of us wanted that to be me, and it wasn't. I angled my chair so I couldn't see the girl anymore.

My recovery was steady, but slow, and both my mother and I clung to every minor improvement. But there was no way I would wake up tomorrow and simply get out of bed on my own. We both knew that.

For this girl, her injury might only be a hiccup in her life, a story to tell friends and lovers as the years passed. For most people, it would be a terrifying one at that. "I couldn't walk. I couldn't walk at all!" Physically, at least, she likely wouldn't be marked.

I was on a continuum, possibly somewhere between this girl and Peter from work. I still didn't know where I would end up.

"I have a good life," Peter had said. And he did. But I also now knew how difficult it was as a quadriplegic to fully participate in daily life. The struggle, the time, the frustration, the patience, the help required to bathe, to dress, to eat, to move, and the problems with bowel and bladder function.

Not long after my accident, my mother and Daniel were visiting me. It had been about a week since I'd almost died, and I was grateful. "It's enough," I'd said, "to be talking to you, here, now, the light coming in through the windows, my mind still okay. It's enough to be alive for." And it had been then, but somehow it wasn't anymore. Even if I had no further recovery, I had to be like Peter. And I would be. I'd cope with the challenges of being quadriplegic and fully re-enter my life.

SEPTEMBER 13

I HOVERED NEAR the baseline, feet shoulder width apart, knees slightly bent, my arms loose, limber, feeling the leather grip, the weight of the racket in my hand. The sun beat down on the open court. Perspiration trickled down my back. I was alert, poised, ready to receive the serve. It came hard and fast. I lunged and swung, my backhand strong, controlled, the ball sailing past my opponent, landing deep in the back corner, right on the line.

"That's game," I shouted. "Game. Set. Match!" Then suddenly I was very thirsty. My mouth was dry; my throat was parched. Water. I needed water. Water!

I jolted awake. Struggled to orient myself: the white room, the side rails of the hospital bed, my body.

My tongue was glued to the roof of my mouth. Thirsty. So thirsty. A large thermal cup of ice water stood on the night table, only about a foot away. But…it was impossible to reach. If only I could return to the dream…to my true self. I pressed the call bell and waited.

But I didn't want to wait. I wanted to get up and fetch the water myself. Like I always had. Not be captive to this worthless body. This was not how I was supposed to be.

The call bell continued to ring.

"Are you awake?" Gary peeked in the doorway.

"Come in," I said relieved someone was here. "Can you bring the water to me? It's on the nightstand."

"Sure, sweetie." Scooping up the pitcher, he placed it on the over-bed table, rolling the table so it was across the bed, and the long straw of the cup was right in front of me.

"I still can't reach it." Now it was just *inches* away. "I need to be higher."

He elevated the head of the bed. "That better?"

I placed my mouth over the straw and the cold water moistened my mouth and throat. Finally. "Can you turn off the call bell? I just needed water. I don't want them in here unless they have to be."

Gary pressed the flashing button on the intercom and settled into a chair beside me. "I got approved for my stress leave today. Four months and then we'll see how I am."

"What?"

"My employee assistance counselor, Joanne, suggested it. She thinks I'm really depleted. That I need time to recover and balance things."

"*Four months?* But you weren't even hurt."

"I did a questionnaire and my stress ratings were off the chart. I've got a lot on my plate, you know? I need to be a good father to Crystal, take care of myself, and come to see you every day. At least during my *scheduled* hours."

I ignored the provocation. I was grateful that my mother had created a visiting timetable so that Gary and Daniel each came separately and they never met.

"How was physio today?" Gary asked, after a few minutes of silence.

"Fantastic. I've gotten more movement back in my left arm. Just over the last few days. Watch this." Eyes fixed on my left hand, I etched the movement in my mind, paralleling the physical movement, as I flexed my left wrist. My hand rose upward slowly, haltingly. I held it briefly at the top, the back of my hand at almost a ninety-degree angle to my forearm, then I released and my hand dropped down. "There." I exhaled, unaware I'd been holding my breath.

"And there's this too." Again I eyed my left hand and forearm where it rested beside me on the bed. Up. Up. Up. The forearm and hand lifted together in a straight plane. Next, I raised my elbow until it hovered about two inches in the air. "And down!" I let go and the arm returned to my side. "I think my shoulder is doing that. Maybe the trapezius. I'll have to ask." A chart that hung in the physiotherapy room depicted all the muscles in the human body, a man's body, both front and back views. I was trying to learn the name of each muscle group, to memorize their shapes and functions as they rolled over joints, creating perfectly synchronized movements. I wanted the chart emblazoned in my mind so I could visualize and help direct and strengthen every new connection, every movement that returned to me.

"That's really great," Gary said, his eyes lighting with his smile.

"Let me try one more." I moved my eyes to my left elbow. Bend. Bend. A jerk. A twitch where it lay on the bed. "The biceps are about the same as yesterday. But at least I can see the elbow move a bit now." That *was* something, but I hungered for more. "My occupational therapist thinks I'm ready to use a power chair. She's going to adapt a joystick so I can drive it. We're going to try it tomorrow."

"That's wonderful. You're getting better every day. That reminds me, I made you something." Gary waved a cloud with scalloped edges made of teal construction paper in front of me. "See what I wrote?"

"The Sky Is the Limit" was inked across the cloud in black marker. The phrase Dr. Davis, my rehab doctor, had used a few days ago when I'd asked about my recovery. There were no guarantees, he'd said, but I was progressing well.

Before the accident, I'd sneered at the motivational posters Gary hung in his office, his Anthony Robbins tapes, and his belief that growing his multi-level marketing business was the key to his future financial success. I'd cringed when he'd tried to unload pot scrubbers or cleaning products on an unsuspecting friend or acquaintance and wondered again what I was doing with him. We had so little in common.

But while the sign he'd crafted was hokey, I didn't feel contempt. Right here, right now, I'd take whatever I could get.

"I'll put it up." Gary ripped a piece of scotch tape from a roll. "How about here?" He indicated a blank space on the wall. "You've got so many cards up already, soon there won't be room for any more."

The wall was festooned with cards from friends, family, coworkers, friends of my mother, my father, my grandmother, and distant relatives I could barely recall. A potted violet, daisies, sunflowers, and two plush teddy bears lined the windowsill while a bouquet of "Get Well" balloons floated in a corner. Overall, the bright colors, the cheery festivity, resembled a child's nursery.

Gary dug into his bag and held up a T-shirt. "This is for you. From my boss, Guy Boucher."

"Why's he giving me a T-shirt?"

"He got it as a souvenir for running a marathon last weekend. He said he ran the marathon for you. And he wanted you to have the shirt to know he is wishing you the best."

"He barely knows me." Guy Boucher was part of the senior management team for my sector. I might have been introduced to him at a management presentation once in the four years I'd worked there. But I knew Gary revered him.

"He knows me. And he certainly knows who you are. I thought it was a tremendous gesture."

"It is thoughtful." And it was, in a way. "But I don't want it. You can keep it."

"Why don't you want it?"

"I just don't. Take it away." I didn't want anyone running in my "honor." It made me feel like I was dead. And I certainly didn't want a reminder of other people's athletic feats. Not when I could barely move and might never be able to again.

Gary frowned and tucked the T-shirt back in his bag. "I'll hold onto it for you. In case you change your mind."

I wouldn't.

"I brought you something else. That I know you'll want. It's in the car."

"What is it?"

"Guess."

"Just tell me."

"I'll give you a hint."

"Come on. It's hard enough…."

"Something that could replace *that*." He pointed to a mounted art poster on the wall.

"I'm not taking it down."

"The other one is much nicer."

"You picked up my *Irises* print?"

"It's a great frame. I had to pay the balance. I don't mind. But just so you know."

"That's okay. How much?"

"A hundred and twenty-five."

"I'll pay you back. Go get it. I want to see it."

"Back in a flash." He whistled out of the room.

I shifted my eyes to the Kandinsky poster on the wall. I'd bought it at an exhibit at the Museum of Modern Art when I went to New York for the first time in April. The trip had been a watershed, a renewal, connecting with friends from university who'd been around even before Daniel. When I'd returned home, I'd started to consider moving back to Toronto to finish my doctorate and after almost two years of procrastination, resumed work on my dissertation proposal. Over the summer, when reading research articles at night, I'd glance at the poster and see the potential for a new life, leaving my government research job, Gary, and most difficult of all, leaving the memory of Daniel behind.

Now I felt a further connection with this print, a deep emotional resonance. *Composition VII*. In the swirls of color and form, the curved lines and objects, the splashes of ivory, ochre, salmon, magenta, and turquoise cut through with sharp lines, a black eye in the turbulence and destruction, I found myself and the possibility of rebirth. This was where I was, from this I would re-emerge.

"Here we go." Gary shuffled into the room. He held up the framed print of Van Gogh's *Irises* so I could view it from my bed.

"It looks really good."

"I forgot picture hooks. I'll bring them tomorrow."

"Thanks."

"No problem. But I'm wiped." He plopped down in the chair, removed his glasses, and rubbed his eyes. The morning sun through the window highlighted his thinning gray hair, his furrowed brow, the creases around his eyes. He looked old. Much older than his forty-six years. No wonder everyone thought he was my father.

"It was a zoo out there," he said.

"Where?"

"In the parking lot, the elevators. Hard to walk through all those people carrying the poster."

"I really appreciate it." Parking. "Um…Gary? I need to talk to you about something."

"Shoot."

"The rehabilitation consultant from the insurance company said there was a problem having both a husband and a common-law husband submitting receipts for visitor parking."

"What's the problem?"

"Why did you say that we were common-law?"

"We are."

"You know we're not."

"You stay over at my place."

"That's not the same."

"Sure it is."

"It's not."

"I don't think it's a big deal."

"It is to me. Anyway, they won't cover your parking."

"But they'll pay for Daniel."

"You can't lie about being in a common-law relationship with me."

"I didn't lie. That's how I see it. Besides, I have plans." He leaned toward me.

"What plans?"

"After you're out of here. I thought we could buy a lot in the country. Somewhere flat. And I'd build a house. All on one floor. All accessible. Just in case. And I'll make a large deck out back, overlooking a garden, and—"

"Stop." My body tensed. "Just stop for a minute. Okay?"

"What?"

"I don't..."

"What?"

"The accident hasn't changed anything. We weren't living together before, and...."

"You don't want to live with me?" The chair grated against the floor as he stood. He gripped the bed rails and bent over, his face inches above mine. "Is that it?"

"Gary." His breath was acrid, suffocating. "Sit down."

He pushed away from the bed and stepped back a few feet. "I don't get this. Do you even want to be together at all?"

"As friends. But I have to focus fully on myself. On trying to get better."

"I thought the accident would make us closer, not push

us apart. Of course, the most important thing is you getting well. But what am I supposed to do?"

"You?"

"I'm just not sure where this leaves me. Without a girlfriend, I guess."

"You'll have to figure that out."

"Do you still want me to come here?"

From the clock, I could see it was nearly nine. "Of course. But I can't talk about this anymore. Martha will be in soon to get me dressed."

"I'll go." He grabbed his jacket. "But I need to think about this, you know? It's thrown me."

After he left, I inhaled deeply, releasing the tightness that had seized my body. How could he think we were common-law? Why would he plan to build us a house? We'd never discussed anything like that before. Was it guilt? His way of taking responsibility?

I wanted no part of it. When I finished rehab, I did not want to return to my previous life.

I'd been so depressed for the past two years: unhappy with Gary and, before him, miserable with Daniel.

Before Daniel and I had separated, the last six months of our marriage had been unbearable, the tension constant between us, as if we were balancing a pane of glass. A slight shift and it shattered, an eruption of cutting words and jagged shards of arguments, both past and present. Daniel was distant, finding fault with me, with our life together. At first, I'd tried complying with his demands: refraining from wearing my glasses out in public, never disagreeing with his point of view in front of others, ensuring I always walked beside and never in front of him.

One day we were wandering through the market and my attention was momentarily drawn to a window display while Daniel was talking about a problem at work.

"See. This is what you always do!" he shouted.

"What?"

"You're always distracted. You were looking at the bookstore. You never listen to me."

"Shhh." I glanced around to see if anyone had noticed his yelling. "I *was* listening. I just saw a book I might want to buy. I was listening the whole time. Test me. I can repeat everything back to you."

"It's what you always do. It's because of your parents. They never paid attention to you. You don't know how to pay attention to anyone else."

We were back on familiar ground. I *had* been listening. But this argument always confused me. I didn't think it was true, but maybe he was right.

"I need some time alone." He shouldered his way through the smiling shoppers as I turned toward home, brushing tears from my eyes.

I couldn't remember the exact catalyst after our argument in front of the bookstore, maybe the way I was washing dishes or a disagreement over which video to rent, but the next time Daniel's anger flared and he screamed, "I feel trapped. I want to leave." I'd agreed. "I think that's best for both of us."

And that's when I should have left Ottawa. But I hadn't.

A couple of months later, Gary and I were driving back from a work meeting in Montreal. "You know I like you," he'd said. "I *like* you, like you."

I'd laughed at his innocence, and he was so positive and kind. "I adore you," he'd once said, and I was overwhelmed by how much I needed this, how much I wanted to be adored. We saw more and more of each other outside of work. Somehow our lives became entwined. I couldn't commit to him, but it was easy to just go along. A stopgap relationship. Days turned to weeks, then to months, and somehow over a year had blurred by.

I'd been a stranger in my own life, but now I was ready. To make decisions and changes, to move forward on my own. I didn't know yet how I would do it or what I would do, but I'd find a way.

I studied the *Irises* print propped against the wall. From where I lay, I glimpsed a purple-blue iris against a muted yellow-green background, the curved edge of a leaf. My last day. Strolling down Bank Street the day before the accident, browsing through shops in the Glebe, returning videos, stopping for coffee, then spying the poster in the window, impulsively buying it, and ordering the frame. An ordinary Saturday. My last full day.

I tried to summon the feeling of walking, the lilt of a step, the dash across the street. But I couldn't recreate it, my memory of movement was gone.

What if I'd known? How would I have used those now-precious hours before everything changed? How guilelessly I'd spent that day, not realizing what I had, what I could lose.

I shifted my eyes to the Kandinsky print. The chaos and confusion. The place where I was now. I refocused on the Van Gogh print. What could I regain? Who could I become?

SEPTEMBER 14

"BRING SUSAN OVER to the plinth," Barb, my occupational therapist, said as Pierre, one of the porters, steered me into the room.

He parked me alongside what looked like a large, rectangular, padded massage table. "Okay, here?" he asked.

"I think this is going to work for you," Barb said, maneuvering a black power chair beside me. "I've modified a grip. Should we give it a try? I'll get someone to give us a hand."

I glanced at the power chair. I was seated in a manual chair, belted at the chest and hips. My arms rested on an acrylic tray, my feet on footrests. How would they ever get me from here to there?

Barb was about my age with long, straight, black hair. She had a slight build and hadn't transferred me before. I hoped someone sturdy would help. This forced trust, this inescapable dependency, made me edgy. What if something went wrong and they dropped me on the floor? Smashed. Shattered. Over.

"This is Harry. He's one of the assistants here," Barb said, introducing a lanky, tall man, blond and bearded. "We'll transfer you to the plinth. Then into the power chair."

So that's how they'd do it. Shifting me from place to place was a puzzle I still hadn't quite figured out. But that sounded safe. Safe enough.

"Comfortable?" Barb asked, once they'd settled me in the power chair. The setup was similar: straps across hips and chest, arms on the wheelchair tray, feet on the footrests. I eyed the modified joystick on the left side. A piece of wood shaped like a capital *T* rose from a black base. The horizontal piece of wood, the top of the *T*, was about five inches long and an inch and a half wide.

"Start by placing your hand over the grip," Barb said.

I lowered my eyes to my left arm so my sight could help guide the movement. Every voluntary motion was like this, all my faculties honed on the execution, like a puppet master, uncertain if the strings were attached.

I lifted my forearm a couple of inches off the wheelchair tray, torqued it slightly to the left, then plopped my open left palm onto the grip, curling my fingers loosely around it. "Okay." I expelled a whoosh of air.

"The middle position is neutral," Barb said. "Push forward to go forward; pull back to reverse. Veer to the left to go left; the right to go right. When you let go or keep it in neutral, the chair will slow down to a stop."

"Okay. I've got it." In my mind I knew what to do. But would I be able to connect to my body, to initiate these meager movements of my wrist and hand, inconsequential just a few weeks ago, but everything now?

"Driving it can be a bit tricky, but I know you can do it. The on/off control is here." She indicated a switch on the arm of the chair, just in front of the joystick. "Harry is working on something in the shop that we can use to build this up, to extend it like a handle, so you can work it yourself. For now, someone will have to turn it on and off for you. But I thought you'd want to start using the chair right away."

"I do."

"Let's give it a try. Is your hand in neutral?"

I looked down. "Yes."

"Okay!" She flipped the switch.

I stared at my hand. Reached deep into my brain to form the idea of the movement. Sent the image down, visualized its flow from my cortex, neuron by neuron through nerves, cell by cell, to excite the appropriate muscle sequence. There! I edged the stick forward, maybe a half an inch. The chair lurched ahead. "Oh no!" I relaxed my hand and wrist and the joystick released, repositioning itself to neutral.

"Try to keep your hand steady. Head toward the door. We'll have more room to practice in the hall."

Again, I eased the control forward, striving to maintain a consistent pressure on the grip to hold the forward position. Stay. Stay. Stay. I imagined my hand and the angle of my wrist cemented to the joystick. Hold. Hold. More smoothly this time, I inched ahead, in a straight line to the wide doorway. "I'm moving! I'm moving myself."

We passed through the threshold into the corridor. "Now shift the stick a little to the right. Just a tiny bit. It's wired to be sensitive to the smallest of movements."

Again, from brain through nerve and muscle fibers, I visualized then enacted the movement. "That's it," Barb said. "Turn. Turn. Now straight on again. Excellent!"

"I turned the corner!" I slowed the chair to a halt. Took

a deep breath. Gazed down the long, quiet hallway. "So now we'll go down there?"

"Yes. Stop just before the end. You can go a little faster if you feel comfortable."

As I nudged the joystick forward, the effort of forcing the movement from my mind to body had eased. The messages were getting through, and my motions were more automatic. I had established a new pattern and the response strengthened with each repetition. Behavioral science: I was like a rat in a Skinner Box, pressing a lever. More confident now, I thrust the stick forward and accelerated. I flashed to childhood bike rides in early spring, after the long winter months, whizzing down the big hill at Gibbons Park, the moist air pungent with freshly thawed soil, with renewal. I remembered the rush, the exhilaration of motion.

Near the end of the hall, I released the joystick and brought the wheelchair to a stop. "That was almost fun."

Barb smiled. "You're doing great. Now. See that?" She indicated a convex mirror, installed in the upper corner where the two hallways intersected. "That allows you to see around the corner. That way you can adjust your speed, be aware of any other people or objects that might be in your way before you turn."

Did every hospital have these mirrors? Other public buildings? I had no idea. The injury had not just radically altered my body but had also changed my perception of the environment. This new body no longer fit in with the world. Even in the accessible space of the rehab center, I'd noted potential obstacles, like the ATM near the elevator. The bank machine was at a low height, appropriate for wheelchair users, but my hand and arm function would have to improve significantly for me to use it. And beyond that? Outside the rehab center, I thought about how impossible everything would be. How…. Stop. I couldn't let myself think about it. I had to focus on this moment. Just this moment. I had to focus on this convex mirror that Barb had pointed out, invisible to me before, that would help me avoid collisions and keep me safe. Here. Now.

"Ready?" Barb asked.

I pushed the stick forward and as the corner approached, flitted my eyes to the mirror, then shifted the joystick a little to the right. I lacked precision, but with a fairly wide arc, I turned into the adjacent corridor.

"Well done. Over the next few days, we'll practice navigating in tighter spaces."

We continued on. About halfway down the hall, I veered to the right to hug the wall as two women, files tucked under their arms, strode briskly toward us. As they neared, I recognized one of the nurses who'd been assigned to me once or twice when Martha had taken a day off. And the other…. No…. It couldn't be, but it was. A little thinner, maybe, but the other woman was Angela. I'd taken a statistics class with her last year.

She was probably doing a psychology internship here, her life persisting on a predictable course since we'd last met. While my life was broken, reduced to this: a halo, a barely functioning body, a prop in a chair.

I couldn't let her see me. Not like this. But I had nowhere to go. No choice but to be on display. My legs trembled with an involuntary spasm. I fought to steady my grip, to keep moving forward.

Then they were upon us. They nodded to Barb and passed at a clipped pace. Their heels echoed on the tiled floor as they kept going, businesslike, purposeful.

Angela had failed to recognize me. Neither of them had even looked my way. I was invisible.

Barb and I reached the end of the hall. I slowed the chair and, in what was already on the cusp of becoming an automatic motion, shifted the joystick to the right and executed the turn.

"You're really getting good at this," she said.

But I didn't care. Seeing Angela had robbed me of any sense of progress. Triumph became tragedy, pride became shame, something became nothing, and that was me. I was nothing.

SEPTEMBER 20

"HEY, SEXY," Jack said as he rolled up in his wheelchair.

I slowed to a halt. Pierre, who was escorting me, pushed the up button on the elevator.

"Hi, Jack," I said.

Jack had a goatee and looked like he was in his mid-thirties. He was balding, burly, and probably fairly short, though I'd never seen him standing. A paraplegic. Complete.

"I'm just coming from physio," he said. "Learning to pop wheelies in my chair so I can get over curbs, shit like that, when I get out."

"How'd it go?"

"Kinda cool. I was the best in the class."

"That's great." The elevator doors opened. "Let me go in, then you can get out first upstairs. I can drive forward pretty well but I'm still not very good at backing up or turning in small spaces. So, it takes me a while to get out of the elevator."

"That's why you got Pierre here to help. Right, man?"

"Sure thing, Jack."

When we reached the second floor, I tugged the handgrip

toward me in an attempt to back out of the elevator, but the chair veered to the left and I got stuck in the corner.

"I told you," I said. The elevator beeped; the doors had remained open too long. I thrust the grip away from me to move forward, but I pushed too hard and rammed into the opposite corner. "No…," I groaned.

"Let me give you a hand," Pierre said. He grasped the control and maneuvered me out of the elevator.

"I'm awful at this."

"Don't worry," Pierre said.

"You'll get the hang of it," Jack said.

"I don't know. My arm still needs to work better so I can control it." I glanced at Jack, his tattooed arms, his gloved hands resting on the wheels of his manual chair. If only I could get my arms—or even my left arm—back, I would be able do so much more.

"What're you up to now?" Jack asked.

"Resting a bit before my next appointment. You?"

"Grab a smoke, then chat with the ladies." He nodded to where the nurses were gathered at the reception area.

In my room, I pulled up to the window. Only about fifteen minutes before the porter would return to take me to physio. Not enough time to be transferred into bed to lie down. I felt a flash of jealousy toward Jack. Paras could transfer themselves with their arms. I could do nothing.

We'd met during my first week at the rehab center when he dropped by my room.

"Hi, I'm Jack." He wheeled toward me. "You're Susan, right?"

"Yeah." I'd seen him in the halls on my way to physio

and OT. But why was he here? I relished my privacy, my single room, so grateful that because we were separated, not divorced, it was covered through Daniel's extended health insurance.

"Thought I'd pop in for a visit."

"I'm pretty tired."

"I won't stay long. Keeps up the spirits to talk to someone. You were in a car accident, right?"

"I was."

"I totaled my bike driving back from a party in the country. Out of nowhere a bird flew into my face. I swerved and crashed right into a brick wall. Never saw the wall. It wasn't there and then it was. What about you?"

I told him the story I'd been telling for almost three weeks. The story that had become my only story.

"A moose?" he said. "That's fucked up."

"I know." I smiled. It *was* fucked up.

"What happened to the driver?"

"Nothing. A few scratches."

"And he was sober? No booze? No weed?"

"Just a freak accident."

"I got to admit, I'd had a few shots. Vodka. Have a taste for it. Like the old man. This the first time you been in the hospital?"

"First time." Then I remembered an overnight stay with Jell-O and ice cream when I was four.

"I was in two summers ago. Not this place. A different hospital. They didn't treat me so good there. I guess I deserved it. I got to tell you, I was a bad man. A really bad man. I think that's why this happened. You know? God telling me it's enough. Time to change my life." His face went blank. "I was in there because I got shot. Right here." He pointed to his lower right abdomen, then yanked up his T-shirt. "See the scar?"

The puckered skin was pink and shiny where the bullet had entered. "That must have been scary," I said.

"It was kind of in the line of duty, you know? Part of the job." He looked down then up again, his face brightening.

"You like dogs?"

"Sure."

"My brother, he has this big place. An old farm in Stittsville. That's where I was, you know, that night? He raises dogs. A whole bunch of them are going to have babies in October. I could get you one if you want."

"Oh?"

"They're real good watchdogs. Pit bulls. Cutest puppies I ever seen. Just let me know and I'll arrange it like that." Jack snapped his fingers. "He's got some Shepherds too. But you got to learn German to have one of them. Sitz. Halt. Shit like that. It's all they understand."

After that, whenever we met, I was friendly and polite.

Jack seemed to believe his injury was a result of fate, a form of punishment, but I didn't. While I tried to avoid thinking about my accident, sometimes I replayed the events of that night. What if we'd stayed home and left the next morning? What if we'd rented a car? A bigger, newer car with air bags? What if I'd insisted we stop for coffee just minutes before? But why waste time considering it? It was a random event with no reason or lesson. It could never be undone.

■ ■ ■

Midnight and I was struggling with sleep, still disrupted by Daniel's visit earlier that evening. One minute he'd say, "Maybe we'll still have kids together someday." Then a few minutes later, he'd tell me he'd just put a down payment on a condo with a bedroom loft. When he was with me, he wanted to escape; but when we were apart, he wanted me back. He'd always been like that. Why had I tolerated it?

I had to stop thinking about him, to steel myself, to focus on recovery.

Gravol. Maybe a couple would help me sleep. I pressed the call bell for the nurse.

A few minutes later, a nurse I hadn't met before entered the room.

"Two Gravol for you, right?" She leaned over me and tugged the cord to turn on the light above the bed.

"I take them crushed with jam. There's some packets on top of the cabinet."

"Who's *that*? She's so pretty." The nurse pointed to the framed picture that Daniel had given me that evening, a photo he'd taken of me seated on a seawall in Portugal in a bright green sundress, smiling, tanned, my hair streaked blonde by the sun, looking vital, vibrant, radiating health.

"That's me."

"*Really?*" The nurse stirred the pills and jam together.

"Can you give me the water?" I sipped the water and tried to swallow the mixture without gagging.

She kept glancing between the photograph and me. "I can see it a bit, especially around the eyes."

"I'm done. Can you turn out the light?"

"Is there anything else I can do for you?"

"No." Just get out.

"Sleep well."

Whenever we met, Jack greeted me with lines like "Hey, sexy" or "How's it going, sexy?" At first, I'd cringed. I was propped in a chair, a lifeless body, the steel halo bolted to my head, caging a face swollen with purple and yellow bruises. With time, though, I tried to be less embarrassed, to accept his kindness. Jack's comments belied an understanding that was beyond that of the nurses and staff and until now even beyond me.

I moved my eyes to the photo and ran my tongue over my chipped bottom teeth, the only damage from the accident I could actually feel. I visualized myself, again in the green dress, strolling down a sunlit street, entering an office building, the elevator to the dentist's office. Waiting in the chair for the procedure to begin, eager to receive the final repair.

SEPTEMBER 24

WEEKENDS IN the rehab center were slow. No physiotherapy, no occupational therapy. Fewer nurses and less urgency. No appointments to keep, so the nurses came to bathe and dress me later in the mornings. I'd insisted my mother take a break on weekends, so she usually arrived around noon so she could feed me lunch, and we could go outside if the weather permitted. Daniel and Gary often stopped in, and occasionally other friends would visit. But I felt a lull, a stillness, a quietness that I hated. I far preferred the rhythm of the weekdays, the rush to my sessions, the sense of purpose, like I was moving forward.

Instead, this Sunday morning was static, like I existed only in a dull, stark, white space. At least I was positioned on my side facing the window and the curtains were drawn. I shifted my eyes to the sky outside, bereft of clouds, and watched the rippling light. The sky was blue, so very blue. How many words could I think of to describe the blueness of the sky? Aqua, azure, aquamarine, Robin's egg blue, baby blue, periwinkle....

"Good morning! Remember me?"

"Yes…David, right?" David was a recent nursing grad. Tall and skinny, with straight brown hair, and slightly protruding blue eyes. He'd been assigned to me on weekend shifts before. I hated having a male nurse, a rare occurrence, but still, it happened.

"Time for your catheter," he said, placing a kit on the bedside table. He depressed the intercom button. "Can I get a hand in here to logroll Susan?"

"Nice day out there today," David said. "It was cool this morning when I biked in, but it's supposed to warm up."

I didn't want to hear about how he'd ridden here on his bike. Shouldn't he know that? Didn't they train the nurses not to say such things to recently paralyzed patients?

After a few minutes, another nurse entered my room. They shifted me onto my back, and the other nurse left. I lay, legs spread, and tried to disconnect, to take myself away… away from the body on the bed, the rustling of David opening a catheter kit. I moved my eyes to my Kandinsky poster and attempted to disappear in the bright hues, the shapes, the contrast, and the formation of lines.

"Oh…looky here…. Someone's got her period!" David said.

"What?"

"See?" He held up a white facecloth dotted with drops of blood. My blood! From my *vagina*! "I'll get a pad," he said. "Back in a flash."

The doctors had told me it would be three to six months before my period returned because of my spinal cord injury. Of all things, *that* was what had come back early. My period was barely even late. It was just over a month since my accident.

Why couldn't this have happened with a female nurse? Why did it have to be David? But, of course, there was nothing I could do.

"Here we are," David said, returning to my room. He held up a monster-sized pad that resembled a diaper. He placed it inside my shorts and pulled them up to my waist, poking and prodding, ensuring everything was in place. "Okey-dokey. You're all set now."

I didn't respond. I couldn't. Humiliation had stifled all my words. Please let this be the last time. Please let me have enough hand function and coordination to do this myself next time.

SEPTEMBER 25

I STARED AT the half-peeled banana on my wheelchair tray. Friend or foe? I'd asked Martha to peel it and place it there. I wanted to try to eat this part of my lunch by myself. Since I'd started driving the power chair, my left arm and hand continued to gain strength and function. In addition to daily occupational therapy and physio, every night now I exercised my left hand and arm: wrist curls, bicep curls, and squeezing a stress ball for grip strength. Even though my movements remained a little shaky, last night I'd been able to perform ten repetitions of each exercise. My left arm really seemed to be coming back to me and I wanted forge ahead, use it to do more things. So today I was determined to tackle the banana, to take at least one bite on my own.

I raised my left arm from where it rested on the joystick and inched it toward the banana. Farther. Just a little farther. Keeping my fingers splayed, I lowered my hand to the bottom part of the banana, still sheathed in skin. Squeeze. Gently squeeze. I had it! I stabilized my elbow on the arm of the chair, contracted my biceps, and slowly brought the banana up... up...aiming for my mouth. The tip of the banana brushed my chin. Cold and mushy against my skin, an aroma of fruity decay. But too low. Too low to reach my mouth. I lifted my elbow and levered my arm like a wing. There. Between the bars of the halo, I pulled my hand toward my mouth…and success! I bit into the sweet, soft, sticky fruit, chewed, and swallowed. My first bite! My arm tremored. I released the muscles and slowly guided the arm back to the tray. A short break, then I'd try once more. I'd practice and practice and maybe if I were lucky, I'd be feeding myself again soon.

A few minutes after Martha cleared away my lunch, women's voices chimed in the hallway accompanied by the patter of synchronous footsteps. They came closer and closer, until just outside my room, abrupt silence, then a rap on the half-opened door.

"Susan?"

"Come in." I wasn't expecting anyone.

Tammy and Robin, friends from work, entered my room. Tammy led the way and Robin shuffled in, a little behind her.

"We brought these for you," Tammy said, holding up a pot of rust-colored mums.

"Thanks so much. You can put them over there, on the windowsill."

Robin stared at me for a moment, then quickly averted her eyes. "How are you feeling?"

"Better. I'm doing better every day."

"That's good." Robin gnawed her lip.

Tammy sat on my bed. "Everyone is thinking about you. Rick and Mark and Nicole said to say hi. Why don't you sit down, Robin?" Tammy pointed to a chair.

"I'm fine like this," Robin said. "Standing." She studied

the wall on the far side of the room. "You sure have a lot of cards up there."

"Sorry we didn't come sooner," Tammy said. "We wanted to wait until...you know...until we were sure you were up for visitors."

"That's okay. How are things at work?"

"Well...." Tammy grinned conspiratorially. "Deidre, you know, the cafeteria manager? She got fired. For that incident at the summer BBQ in July."

"What happened again?" I asked. "I don't remember."

"She and the security guard got caught having sex on the kitchen floor. Helga from HR saw them when she went in to get more hot dog buns." Tammy snorted. "What a—"

"Tammy," Robin said. She was clutching her throat.

"Tammy! I can't breathe. I have to get out of here." She staggered out of the room.

"I'll go check on her," Tammy said.

A few minutes later, Tammy returned. "Robin says she's sorry. She was in a halo when she was fourteen because she had scoliosis. It freaked her out to see one again."

"Is she okay now?"

"She's sitting by the nurses' station. They gave her some orange juice. She almost fainted."

"Oh."

"I think we'd better go. But we'll come back another time. Soon. Okay?"

No, they wouldn't. Neither of them would ever be back. I knew that. Was this how things were going to be? People falling out of my life because of my injury, because it was too hard for *them*?

113

I was irritated at Robin and her fainting spell. I understood being in a halo as a teenager had been traumatic for her, but I was paralyzed! It was a little different.

I wished they hadn't come. Even prisoners, at least the ones in movies, had the right to approve their visitors, and they always knew when they'd be coming in. No surprises.

Stuck here, I was like a zoo animal. During the day, people could come and go as they pleased.

Outside my family and close friends, seeing others was hard. Harder than I thought it would be.

Almost two weeks ago I'd been terrified that Angela from my statistics class would notice me in the hall and then startled when she hadn't even registered my presence. With Tammy and Robin, I'd wanted to be seen; as their friend, as someone known; not as a monstrosity in a chair capable of inducing panic. I wished it didn't matter, that it didn't hurt, but it did. I could feel the darkness edging toward me, threatening to engulf me, making me want to claw at myself, to scream, to snarl at the horror I'd become.

But I wouldn't. I couldn't give in to despair.

■ ■ ■

The winter I was fifteen I'd refused to wear a winter coat. Instead, every day I dressed in a loose-fitting, old, black sweater, jeans, and cowboy boots. No jacket, no gloves, no scarf. I'd longed to be completely self-reliant, to prove that nothing could touch me, not the frigid temperatures, the sleet, the bitter wind, the ice, or the snow. I'd willed myself not to feel the cold. And I didn't. Through ruthless determination, I hadn't felt a thing.

I had to recapture some of that resolve now. I couldn't be undone by my damaged body or by others' reactions to it.

Everything was fluid since my accident—fluid and constantly shifting. My life had fractured: between my body and mind, my before and after self, how others viewed me and how I saw myself. Like gazing into a kaleidoscope, with each rotation, each experience, the shards tumbled together in ever-changing ways. But I needed something to hold onto, some of that insular determination I'd had at fifteen to endure anything, so I could create, no matter how small, some constancy of self.

SEPTEMBER 29

"PUSH AGAINST my hand," Sheila, my physiotherapist, said. She reached down and placed her palm on the outside of my left thigh where I lay outstretched on my back on the treatment plinth. I imagined making an angel in the sand and with all my force opened my leg to the side.

"Good work, Susan. That's definitely getting stronger. Let's do ten reps."

I concentrated and repeated the movement. Ten. Nine. Eight....

"Very nice," Sheila said. "Let's try your other leg."

Her touch was warm against the skin of my right thigh. I shut my eyes and tried to connect to my hip, to locate the muscles in my mind, and then I thrust my right leg sideways.

"I felt it move!"

"That's fantastic," she said. "Try again."

Again, I moved the leg, haltingly, sensing the drag of my heel against the vinyl surface of the table. Push. Push.

"There!"

"You moved at least four inches that time. Tomorrow I'll measure the angle so we can track your progress. Nicely done."

"I can't believe it. I couldn't move it at all yesterday. Every day there's something new."

"Like every day is Christmas." Sheila smiled. "I'm going to get the weights. Be right back."

I bent my left leg at the knee, my foot flat on the plinth until it reached almost ninety degrees, then straightened it. I bent and straightened my left arm at the elbow. Curled my left wrist, then released it, made a fist then opened my left hand and wiggled the fingers. Flexed and pointed my left foot. Up and down. Up and down. So much movement. And now the right leg too!

I closed my eyes and visualized myself upright, striding, swinging both arms. Then lying like I was now but on a beach. The cadence of the waves washing ashore, the warm sand cradling my body, the gentle breeze, the briny air. Then wading in, buoyant, floating, the turquoise sea, the azure sky.

■ ■ ■

I thrust the joystick forward and exited through the main doors of the rehab center. Outside on my own! I stopped a few meters from the entrance and inhaled the crisp earthiness of the air. A light breeze grazed my cheeks. The afternoon September sun warmed my face, cupping it like a gentle hand.

I wheeled along the path that crossed the grounds. Two older men and a middle-aged woman clustered by an ashtray chatting and laughing as they puffed on cigarettes. They had undergone partial leg amputations; their prosthetic legs were strapped to the back of their chairs. In physiotherapy, I'd seen them learning how to walk with artificial limbs. They practiced in the gym. Other than a slight hesitation in their gait, fully clothed, they appeared completely "normal."

As I neared, all three craned their necks. Their eyes bored into me. I wanted to shout, "Stop looking at me!"

I sped up, moving further along the walkway, and parked in a secluded spot by one of the flowerbeds where a few roses clung to withering branches. At the other end of the building, another trail led to a wooded area where Jack rolled along, a chubby blonde woman in a fuchsia tracksuit strolling beside him.

Jack never had visitors. His mother was old, practically blinded by glaucoma, so she couldn't make it in. She prayed for him, he'd said, and they spoke on the phone. I'd overheard their calls. Jack on the pay telephone by the nurses' station, his voice angry and insistent, his words a mixture of English and French. He had a brother too but hadn't offered an explanation for his absence.

I was happy to see him with this woman now. They veered toward the trees and disappeared from sight. A few seconds later, a familiar trio emerged from the same path.

Arms and legs pumping in unison, they marched by the rehab center then turned, heading to the far side of the health center campus. I'd seen them before from the window of my room. Every afternoon, promptly at two-thirty, they passed by: the man always in the center, a woman at each side. They were similar in age, height, and shape: short and squat, in their mid-sixties. Today, as always, they wore matching outfits: tan caps and long-sleeved green plaid shirts tucked into twill cotton khakis.

I found their constancy, their predictability, soothing but

also surreal, like a fleeting image in a Fellini film. Were they triplets? Had the man married one twin, getting two wives in the bargain?

"Susan?"

I turned my chair. My mother walked toward me.

"Martha told me you'd come out here. What a beautiful day." She settled on one of the benches.

"What's in the bag?"

"Chicken fingers from the hospital cafeteria." She opened a container. "They're actually really good."

"Can I have one?" This was the first time since the accident that food had appealed to me. Until now, I'd eaten only for function: bran cereal and prune juice to encourage my bowels to return; yogurt and milk to help my fractures heal.

I lifted my left hand from the wheelchair tray and opened it. I fed myself every meal now, eating by hand or using an adapted spoon with a built-up handle that was easier to grip. I was slow and messy, a towel draped around my upper body like a bib. But the more I did it, the better I would be. My mother placed the chicken in my hand. I curled my fingers loosely around it, lifted my elbow, and levered my arm. Between the bars of the halo, I drew my hand toward my mouth and took a bite. "It's delicious," I said.

"Try it with the honey mustard sauce." My mother dipped the chicken in a second, smaller container and handed it to back me.

Again, I repeated the movements. Grasping with my hand, levering my arm, bending my elbow. And then an explosion of tastes hit my tongue—sweet, spicy, salty. I felt like I'd discovered flavor for the first time. "This is really good!"

119

"I'll bring some more tomorrow for lunch. They have other things too."

"I guess I'm finally getting tired of the food here."

"That's a good sign," My mother said and dabbed her lips with a paper napkin. "Do I have anything on my face?"

"No."

She fished a tube of lipstick from her purse and began applying it. Perfectly groomed. Every hair sprayed into place. Even when I was growing up and she'd downed at least a mickey of vodka every night, she'd been careful with her appearance. In the mornings getting ready for work, she'd swig antacid and use eye drops to clear the redness before putting on makeup and curling her hair.

She squinted at me. "I was wondering, honey, if you'd like me to pluck your eyebrows. I brought my tweezers today, just in case."

"I don't care about my eyebrows. Why were you even looking at them?"

"I just noticed. That's all."

"It's the last thing I'm worried about."

"Let me know if you change your mind."

"I have to get to physio. Are you coming to my session?"

"I'll be there in a minute. I'm going to have a quick cigarette."

■ ■

After dinner, I met Jack in the corridor.

"Hey! Saw you out catchin' some rays today," Jack said. "Good day for it."

"The weather's been pretty warm."

"My girlfriend—well, my ex—and I were out for a bit too."

"I saw you. Did you have a good visit?"

"Yeah. Sherry's the mother of my daughter Trina. She's going to bring her next time. She wanted to make sure I looked okay. Didn't want to scare the kid. First time she's seen me."

"I'd better go. I'm meeting someone downstairs."

"Your boyfriend?" Jack asked with a grin.

"My husb…ex-husband."

"He didn't leave you because of this, did he?"

"No. We're still friends. Like you and Sherry."

"You got any kids?"

"No."

"Guess how many kids I got, besides Trina?"

"How many?"

"Eleven."

"Eleven? That's a lot."

"I was pretty wild back in the day. Eye for the ladies. Trina's the only one I see. Like to help them out when I can."

I placed my left hand on the joystick. "I'd better get going."

"I got something to show you." Jack fingered a gold chain at his neck. "See this?"

"It's very nice."

"Fourteen karat. Sherry brought me some jewelry today. All gold. Necklaces and bracelets and shit. If you want anything, let me know. I'll give you a real good deal."

"Thanks. I'll think about it."

"They're not hot."

"No…no…. It's just I don't really wear gold. Only silver. I'm kind of allergic to gold."

"That's too bad. If I get any silver stuff, I'll let you know."

■ ■ ■

Downstairs, I parked near the doors. The lobby was vacant. Dim, fluorescent lights flickered behind the reception desk and pierced the silence with a high-pitched electric whine. So different from the bustle of the daytime, patients and staff flowing in and out, lineups at the snack bar, volunteers at tables selling raffle tickets for charity. I felt edgy and alert, as if I'd crept into an old, abandoned house at night. I hoped Daniel would arrive soon.

The main doors parted. There was a rush of cool, damp air as a woman pushed a child using a wheelchair into the foyer. She shook her umbrella and attended to the boy. His head cocked to one side and he grumbled as she unzipped his jacket. "I'll get this right off and then we can go and see the doggies," she said. He looked about ten. I figured they were here for Pet Therapy night. I'd never gone.

The doors opened again, and Daniel strode into the lobby wearing a beige trench coat and carrying a soft, tan leather briefcase in one hand. I preferred how he'd dressed when we were students, usually in T-shirts or a sweater and jeans. But this was his uniform now: wool suits, crisply pressed shirts, and silk ties.

"Over here." I wheeled toward him.

"This is a nice surprise. What're you doing down here?"

"I got bored in my room so I thought I'd come to meet you."

"Should we go up? I only have about half an hour, but I picked up something today and wanted to bring it to you. I can stay longer tomorrow."

The woman and her son waited by the elevator.

"Hi," I said, as we joined them.

"Hello," the woman said. "Wet night out there." She nodded to Daniel.

"Sure is," he said, as the elevator doors opened. "After you."

The woman guided her son to one corner, and I wheeled in beside him. As the elevator rose, the boy squealed. He grabbed my right arm where it lay flaccid on the wheelchair tray. His fingers, cold and wet from the rain, clutched my wrist.

"Stop it!" I said. His fingernails clawed at my skin. He yanked. "My arm. Daniel. Help." My voice strangled in my throat.

Daniel pried the boy's fingers free and stood beside me, creating a barrier between the boy and me.

"Leave that girl alone," the woman said to her son. When we reached the second floor, she turned to Daniel. "Sorry about that."

"That was awful," I said, when we got back to my room. "He could have wrenched my arm right out of the socket."

"His mother should have been watching him more closely. But he's just a kid. I'm sure he wasn't trying to hurt you."

"He could have hurt me. Badly. What if you weren't there?"

"I was. And you're okay."

As he rummaged through his briefcase, my thoughts turned to the boy, how he'd seized my arm, limp and lifeless on the tray. Daniel didn't know what it was like to be so easily harmed.

"I got you this." He withdrew a CD. "It's a collection of classical music. You should have something decent to listen to. Enough of that moody Leonard Cohen."

"I like Leonard Cohen."

"This is better. I'll put it on for you before I go." He loaded the CD in the player. "I'll see you tomorrow." He grabbed his case and headed out the door.

I wasn't familiar with the first piece, but immediately recognized the second as the initial bars of *Für Elise* echoed through the room. When I was a teenager, taking piano lessons, it had been one of my favorites. One I had actually practiced. I closed my eyes and listened, imagining my fingers hovering over the keys, plucking the single notes, striking the chords. Just a few months ago, I'd considered buying a keyboard, taking lessons again, but this time I'd really commit myself. I'd practice and practice. I'd become good.

My left arm and both my legs tremored with spasms.

Rain sheeted against my window. Even over the music, I could hear it. My eyes flitted to my right arm. Now, danger lurked everywhere, not just in dark alleys, crouched behind bushes, in cars with strangers, or alone on the streets at night. Now, even a young child was a threat, and I couldn't protect myself.

Mozart's Requiem thundered through the speakers. Daniel was always confident he knew what was best. Don't tuck your hair behind your ears. Stand up straight.

Even here, even now, he'd decided what music I should listen to.

But I wanted to hear Leonard Cohen, not Mozart.

I moved to the intercom to call a nurse to change the

music and then stopped. Maybe I could use my left arm to do this on my own. I pivoted my chair and headed to the cupboard. Grasping the lever, I rotated it slightly, tugged, and swung open the wooden door.

The key to the drawer that held my CDs and tapes lay on a shelf just above the height of my shoulder. I lifted my arm, thrust it forward, and seized the large plastic key holder. My arm trembled as I aimed the key toward the lock in the center of the drawer. I concentrated, tried to fit the key into the small opening, but my hand was unsteady. I rested it on my wheelchair tray for a few seconds. I took a deep breath, raised my arm again, lined up the key with the opening, and inserted it.

I turned the key until I heard the click of the lock, shifted my hand to grip the handle of the drawer, and slid it open. Near the top of the pile was the Leonard Cohen tape.

I wheeled to the bedside table and reached up to the portable stereo to turn off the CD. I slipped in the tape and pressed the play button.

"Everybody Knows" filled the room.

OCTOBER 2

KYLE, ONE OF the physio assistants wheeled me up the ramp and positioned me in the center of the base of the treadmill. "Ready to roll?" he asked.

"I guess so." I was nervous, but excited. What would happen? What would work?

My physiotherapist, Sheila, jumped on the treadmill and checked the harness that she'd belted me into a few minutes earlier.

"Feel comfortable?" she asked.

"I'm good."

"Let's get started." Sheila clipped straps from the harness to a pulley system attached to a metal bar that ran lengthwise above the treadmill. Another physiotherapist, Heather, who was part of the body-weight support research team, joined Sheila on the treadmill platform behind me.

"Ready?" Sheila asked.

"Yes."

"Okay, Kyle. Let's go."

Kyle turned the crank on the pulley system and, while Sheila and Heather spotted me, I rose from the chair until I was suspended above the treadmill upright in the harness, my feet touching the platform. Heather wheeled the chair back down the ramp and sat down at the desk.

I took in the room from this new height. Ceiling, floor, walls. I was now standing on the treadmill in the midst of all this space. Supported, but on my own two feet. And I felt good. Really good. Not dizzy. Not nauseated. Just ready. Ready to begin.

"How much weight should we take off?" Kyle asked Sheila.

"Let's start with seventy-five pounds. About half of Susan's body weight."

"Because of the halo," I said. "It adds about fifteen pounds." I reached out my left hand and grasped the rail of the treadmill. "Look! I can hold on."

"That's great," Sheila said. She hopped off the treadmill and squatted by my right leg. "Ready to start?"

"Yes."

"Set it at point one miles per hour, Kyle." Sheila held my right foot with both her hands. The belt of the treadmill slowly began to move. "Okay," she said, "step with your left foot."

I stepped. I simply stepped. My left leg seemed to remember how to walk. The knee bent. The foot found its way. I couldn't believe it. "Wow!"

"Fantastic, Susan. Good work. Now, let's try the right." Sheila guided my right leg and foot through the motion of a step. The foot and leg were rigid, so bending and straightening the knee and pushing off with the foot was like moving a hundred-pound leg made of steel.

I concentrated, trying to send energy into my right leg and foot to help Sheila as she moved it, but I wasn't sure if I was making any difference.

"I think we can go up to point two miles per hour," she said.

We continued for two more minutes. I stepped with my left and fought to force my right leg through the movement.

"Let's take a break." They lowered me back into my chair. My right leg bobbed up and down with a spasm.

"Put your left hand on your right knee and press down," Sheila said. "That will put pressure on your foot. The weight bearing helps calm the spasm."

I tried it. "It worked!"

Sheila wiped perspiration from her forehead. "I'm not sure if that was harder for me or for you." She grabbed my thermal cup. "I'll go get us some water."

I was exhausted but exhilarated. Walking! Slow, staggered, and assisted, but walking! The left leg was good. I just needed the right to get better. I felt electrified. Maybe someday I'd really be walking again on my own! Free of the chair! Free of paralysis!

I was so lucky to be part of this study. The body-weight support-system training was new for the rehab center too. I was their first research subject. By having me walk on the treadmill with reduced body weight, they were trying to stimulate the walking reflex that everyone has from birth. The hope was that this would help me learn to walk again, despite the injury. Apparently, there had been promising results with cats in Sweden or somewhere in Europe, but I was one of the first humans to try it.

"Have some water." Sheila held the cup under my mouth so I could sip water through the straw. Cold. Icy. Delicious. She grinned. "Ready for another go?"

OCTOBER 4

BARB, MY OCCUPATIONAL therapist, placed a handgrip tester in my left hand. "Squeeze as hard as you can."

I stared at my hand and focused, trying to channel energy from my brain to the nerves and muscles in my hand. I grasped the two metal handles together with as much force as I could. I grunted. "How did I do?"

Barb read the gauge and jotted the number in my chart. "We have to repeat this two more times to get your score."

Again, I gripped the handles with all my strength, and she recorded the number. "Just once more," she said.

My entire arm was trembling. I squeezed for the third time. Harder.... Harder.

Barb took the handgrip tester from me and returned it to its case.

I shook out my hand to release the tension. "How did I do?"

"Remember at first you could barely move the needle? Well, you've even improved since last week. Now you're consistently measuring at about eight kilograms."

"What would be normal?"

Barb consulted a set of tables on a sheet. "For a thirty-year-old woman, non-dominant hand grip is usually around nineteen kilograms. You're nearly halfway there." She checked her watch. "We have about ten minutes left. Feel like a game of checkers?"

"Sure."

"I'll go get the board."

My father stood in the doorway, eyes glancing furtively around the room. "Hey, Dad," I called. "Over here."

"Hi, honey." He joined me at the table.

"I wasn't expecting you until later this afternoon."

"I got an early start and the traffic was pretty good. The nurses told me where you were. It's okay that I came down here?"

"Mom comes to my sessions all the time. They don't mind."

"That's good." He shuffled his feet.

"You can sit down beside me. It's okay."

"Good. Good." He took a seat.

"Here's Barb." She came toward us carrying a checkerboard.

My dad rose from his chair and extended his hand. "I'm Susan's father."

"Good to meet you," Barb said. "She's doing remarkably well. You must be proud of her."

"Of course." He nodded. "Of course."

She stood the oversized checkerboard upright on the table. It was stabilized by a stand and the squares and pieces were covered with Velcro. Large loops on the checkers made them easier to hold. Barb and I had played once before, and

I had moved five pieces before my arm fatigued. Today, I wanted to do better.

"We were just going to have a game of checkers," Barb said. "Why don't the two of you play? Susan has a few minutes of her session left."

"Does this work the same as regular checkers?" my dad asked when Barb left.

"Yes. Do you want to be black or red?"

"I'll take black." He moved the first piece.

I focused, willing my arm to extend forward and my fingers to grab one of the pieces. Coordinated muscle movements were hard and my triceps were still very weak. My arm tremored slightly, but I clasped the piece and moved it one square. "There." I exhaled from the effort.

"You left yourself open." My father captured one of my red pieces. "One to nothing. Your turn."

I scrutinized the board. Which of my checkers would be easiest to reach? I concentrated and moved another piece ahead one square.

"Got you again." Grinning, he plucked another of my red pieces from the board.

"It's not a competition. It's therapy for my arm."

"I know *that*. Just trying to make it interesting."

Once more, I aimed my arm at the board and attempted to seize a piece, but the arm began to shake with a spasm. "I'm too tired to play. Let's just go back to my room."

"Whatever you want, sweetheart."

I placed my hand on the joystick of the power chair and backed away from the table, circled, and headed toward the door. My father followed behind.

"Should I push you?" he asked.

"I can drive myself pretty well. My arm is much better than it was."

When we reached the elevator, I positioned myself parallel to the doors in front of the large button. I lifted my left arm, flung it sideways, and hit the button with the back of my hand. A new skill. When the call bell lit up, I swiveled the chair to face my father. He was staring at the floor numbers across the top of the elevator, tapping his foot.

"Jesus, these elevators are slow."

"The doors have to stay open longer. Most of the people here need extra time to get in and out."

"Right." He flushed. "That's good, you know, that they operate like that."

In my room, I parked by the window.

My father paced.

"You can sit down, Dad. Mom left a magazine here. Why don't you read for a while? I'll rest."

"Whatever works for you, honey." He picked it up and plopped down in a chair.

I pivoted the wheelchair to look outside. Hospital staff and visitors were milling about on this mild fall day with jackets slung over their shoulders. Some sat together on wooden benches, smoking or eating packed lunches, chatting and laughing.

Why hadn't my dad noticed how well I drove the power chair? And that I'd pressed the elevator call button on my own? When he'd last been here, I could barely use my hand.

My stomach ached with a familiar emptiness. For as long as I could remember, I had been under his radar. Even as far back as when I was three years old and lived with my parents in an apartment in my grandparents' house, the house my mother had grown up in. My mom worked, my dad attended teacher's college, and I spent my days with my grandma. One day, my grandma bought a set of fridge magnets at the grocery store: purple grapes, red apples, oranges, bananas, ladybugs, and butterflies. I loved them, their splashes of color, their tiny, perfect shapes. Playing with them, I found that by placing one magnet above and one below a tea towel, their magnetic points touching through the thin fabric, I could guide the bottom magnet with one hand hidden under the towel, and it would appear as if the top magnet were scooting across the surface on its own.

I'd discovered magic! With my grandma's help, I planned a show for my parents and grandpa when they returned home at the end of the day. All afternoon I'd practiced, perfecting the performance, using the piano bench as my stage.

"Ta-da!" I'd shouted, at the end of the act. "Magic!"

"But that's just how magnets work," my dad had said, peering over his newspaper. "There's nothing special about that." I'd screwed up my eyes, trying not to cry, and fled to my room. My mom had followed, rubbed my back while I curled into a ball on my bed, squeaking out tiny sobs. "He's just tired, honey. He's had a long day," my mom said. "Grandma, Grandpa, and I thought your show was wonderful. You should be really proud." But it hadn't helped. Even remembering it now, it hurt. Why didn't I matter?

Another memory surfaced. When I was around twelve, about a year after my parents had separated, I was having lunch one Saturday with my dad at a pizza parlor. Kathryn

134

wasn't there. She was staying with her babysitter, something she'd been doing more and more, even though Glenda wasn't paid on weekends. Glenda had a houseful of older children and always said, "We all love having her here."

As we waited in silence for our food to arrive, I wondered if Glenda took Kathryn home with her because she *knew*, knew the secret that I was going to try to tell my dad now.

He gulped his draft and jiggled his knee up and down under the table, restless, like he couldn't wait to bolt down his pizza and beer to be free to go. I sipped my frosted mug of root beer, gathering the courage to speak.

When the pizza arrived, my dad signaled to the waitress for another beer, grabbed a slice, and dug in. Head low over his plate, strings of hot cheese trailing from his beard, he shoveled it in.

I needed to interrupt his gobbling. I *had* to do this, had to tell him what was going on. "Dad. Daddy." He was so hard to reach as if he were tuned into an eternal hockey game with no commercial breaks. *"Dad!"*

"What, honey?"

"Mommy came home really drunk last night."

"Are you sure?"

"Her friends had to carry her in, put her to bed."

"Sometimes that happens. Nothing to worry about."

"Daddy?"

"What?"

"I think mom drinks too much, like…like an alcoholic." There. I'd finally said it.

"No. She's a social drinker. Like me."

"But she drinks every night, and on Saturdays and

Sundays she drinks and sleeps all day. Sometimes, we can't even wake her up. I make us a box of macaroni and cheese or heat up cans of ravioli, but I really don't know how to cook."

My dad frowned and shook his head. "It's not so bad for you to be independent. Your mom works hard, like me. She's exhausted at the end of the week. Booze is like medicine. It relaxes people. Don't worry. Your mother's fine." He emptied his glass. "All set?"

I knew the discussion was over. I couldn't contradict him. Disagreeing or "lippiness," as he termed it, wasn't allowed. Or else. The threat of violence always hung in the air. I was on my own.

So why now? Why did I want him here now?

"Hey, Dad." I turned my chair to face him. "Remember, when I was little, you'd take me fishing at Grandma and Grandpa Jeffreys' cottage?"

"Of course I do, honey." He set down the magazine. "That was a great place they had there."

"It was fun." I could see us now on the clear, calm lake in the silver aluminum motorboat. My dad casting near the shoreline—toward the fallen trees, their branches protruding from the water like skeletons—because the bass were attracted to the shade of the logs. My pole dangling from the front of the boat where I sat reading, my outstretched legs resting on a cooler that held sandwiches and cans of ginger ale for me and beer for my father. He was a peaceful, almost gentle man on the water, so different from the one at home who flew into purple rages, hurling plates of spaghetti at the kitchen wall. The one whose explosive shouting had woken me at night when I was four and five years old, compelling me to scurry from my bed and fling my small body in front of my mother and cry, "Don't hurt my mommy. Don't hurt my mommy."

"Maybe if I get well enough, you and I could go up north and go fishing again."

"That's a great idea. I'd love that. I really would."

"I should probably get some rest now before my appointments this afternoon."

"I could do with a nap myself. I'm pretty beat after the drive. When should I come back?"

"Uh…." I had a physiotherapy session later, my third trial on the body-weight support system, my walking training. But I didn't want him there, couldn't take the risk. "Around six-thirty. I'm done everything by then."

■ ■ ■

I glanced at the clock. My dad would be here soon. A few minutes earlier I'd buzzed the nurse to clear away my dinner tray and remove the stain-splattered towel draped across my chest like a bib. Even though I could now feed myself, I was messy, and I didn't want my father to see me eating. Last time he'd visited, and I'd explained that I needed to be fed when my lunch had arrived, he'd gone to find my mother who he said was "better at that sort of thing."

Promptly at six-thirty, he ambled in carrying a can of diet cola. His face was ruddy, and his thinning hair and salt-and-pepper beard and mustache looked like they'd been shellacked with black shoe polish.

"Did you do something to your hair?"

He grinned. "Touched it up with a dab of hair color for

men. I comb it in. It's not dye, just gets the gray out. Used it on my beard and moustache too. Looks natural, don't you think?"

"Sure."

"Shaves a few years off. Don't want the nurses thinking your dad's an old man. Did I ever tell you about the lady in Florida who thought I was Burt Reynolds?"

"Yes. So, what else did you do this afternoon?"

"Just relaxed from the drive. Had a few beers, watched some TV. Took a snooze." He sipped his pop. "Spiked it with a little rum." He winked.

"Take it easy, okay? I'm pretty sure you're not supposed to bring alcohol in here."

"Just takes the edge off. My tooth is still a little sore." He rubbed his jaw. "I had a cavity filled yesterday. And I told the dentist not to use any freezing."

"Why did you do that?"

"It's silly really, but…well…I thought if you could be so brave, then…I know it's not the same…but that I could stand it…." He sat down and looked away, took a gulp of his drink.

"That must have hurt." My voice was gravelly. He'd thought of me. Done it for me.

"It's nothing compared to what you're going through, but…anyway…." He looked up. "How was your afternoon?"

"I had a good physiotherapy session on the treadmill. You remember the research study to help me walk again? They move my right leg through a step. I can step with my left leg on my own. I walked for four minutes altogether. With breaks."

"That sounds terrific. You're doing really well."

"It takes a long time. But it's been almost a month since I saw you. I *have* changed a lot since then."

"Just keep it up. I can't wait to tell my parents. They want a full report when I get back." He bent forward and rested his elbows on his knees. "You know, my dad fell apart when I called to tell them what happened to you. Wept like a baby. Had to give the phone to my mother."

"I know." He kept telling me how upset my grandfather had been as if it were a precious gift, a sign of real caring. My grandparents had sent me a fruit basket, and when I spoke to my grandmother, my mother holding the phone to my ear, she'd said, "Granddad is very glad your father has been coming to see you." They expected so little of each other. Even I wasn't surprised that my granddad had been distraught and that my father visited me. After all, I'd almost died. I was paralyzed. What more could it take?

"We're going to drive to London at Thanksgiving," my dad said. "Take my parents out for dinner. Saves my mom cooking a big turkey. There's a place near Thamesford that they like. Reasonable prices too. I guess your mother will be here with you?"

"Lisa's going to come down too, so it should be fun. You remember my friend Lisa? From university?"

He nodded and settled back in his chair. "It's great to see you, honey. Kind of great to get a few days off work too. Did I tell you about the other Special Ed teacher in my department at school? The fat one who's driving me nuts?"

"I think so."

"She's always nagging at me, trying to organize committees, improve parent-teacher relations, all this horseshit—just

139

to make herself look good. Then she complains I'm not pulling my weight. One of those phony, do-gooder personalities. You know the type?"

"Um…I guess."

"I'm not having any part of it. Just want to put in my last few years with the board, then retire. Getting into the politics of the place isn't my style. I want to focus on the kids in my class and get the hell out of there at three each day. Though I got to say, the principal has been really good to me ever since you got hurt. Told me to take off as much time as I need. So, you know what I've been doing?"

"What?"

"Taking some days off here and there. Going down to the track, having a couple of beers. Never bet more than twenty bucks. I know my limit. Helps me let off some steam. Get away from that fat bitch for a while. Of course, some of the time, I come down here to see you. But I'm not going to come every weekend, so I figure why not? I can use the extra days off too." He drained the rest of his drink.

Out. I wanted him out. Just out. "You must be getting hungry, Dad. Maybe you should go?"

He looked startled.

"Mom said the two of you were going out for dinner. She's down in the smoking lounge if you want to go get her?"

"You're okay here by yourself? I can wait to eat."

"I'm tired. I've had a long day. You go ahead."

"Whatever's best for you." He reached over and patted my arm. "I'll drop by in the morning before I hit the road. Love you."

Right.

I wheeled to the window. Dark by seven o'clock now, I wanted to see if I could make out the stars against the night sky. I was so relieved to be alone, to be free of my father. How often I'd felt that way when I was younger. I was always happier away from my parents, the only way I could have space for myself.

The therapists and nurses often commented on my strength, my resolve to get better. Maybe in some ways, my parents had helped me. I'd had to rely on myself. Maybe that's why I was so resilient.

When I was younger, I used to tell my friends that my parents should never have had children, that that was the problem. As if it were an explanation, a kind of excuse, as if the way they treated me wasn't personal. But my mother had changed; she really was here for me now. My father wasn't, probably couldn't be. He was doing his best, but it wasn't enough.

Should I have confronted him? Told him how painful it was to hear that he used my accident as an excuse to take time off work? That fathers who really loved their children didn't do that? That they'd want to be with their daughter as much as possible, even if it was hard?

But how did I alter a lifetime of practice? With my father, protests were ignored or punished. Silence was safety. And so somewhere early on, I'd lost my voice.

Now the rules of survival were different. I had to assert myself. I was trying to speak up more and more but I had to persist, unlearn what was reflexive, because along with my body, everything else had also changed.

I gazed out the window and studied the sky. Dark clouds shifted to reveal a luminous moon and countless scattered stars. If I kept looking, maybe I'd see a falling star.

OCTOBER 6

MY ROOM WAS DIM. Even with the curtains parted, the weak light leaving the overcast sky barely penetrated the window. I dozed in bed. The session on the body-weight support system that afternoon had been strenuous. I'd walked for five minutes without stopping. It was my longest time on the treadmill so far! I wanted to be well rested for tomorrow. Lisa was coming from Toronto to spend Thanksgiving weekend with me. It was something to look forward to. Like everyone else, I was going to have a holiday.

Three knocks at my door. The sudden blaze of overhead lights stung my eyes, I blinked. Short, quick steps and a youngish man in a white lab coat appeared at the side of my bed.

"Susan? Susan Mockler?" He tapped his pen against a clipboard nestled in the crook of his arm. "I'm Dr. Pinkus." He thrust a hand toward me and then shoved it in his pocket when I didn't respond. "I'm here to examine you."

"What?"

"Didn't they tell you I'd be coming by?"

"No."

"I'm an orthopedic resident doing a two-week rotation here. I have to examine all the spinal cords. You're my last one. And the only Brown-Sequard."

"Can't this wait until next week?"

"I told Dr. Davis I'd be done by the end of today. I'm running a little behind."

His timing was odd, almost six o'clock on the Friday of a long weekend. I scanned the hospital identification card hanging by a chain from his neck. It was legitimate. "Okay, but I'm tired. I don't want it to take too long."

"It's just a neuro exam. Less than half an hour. I'm very efficient."

My last neurological exam had been a week ago. Maybe I'd have improved since then.

Dr. Pinkus assessed the strength in each limb. My right arm remained useless, but when I straightened my left elbow against the resistance of his hand, my triceps seemed stronger than before.

"Interesting." He jotted down notes and numbers and shook his head. "C1/C2 fractures. You're very lucky. Most people with injuries above C3 die. Right on the spot. Those that survive usually need mechanical respirators to breathe. For the rest of their lives." He sounded like he was reciting from a textbook.

"I know." I was sick of being told I was lucky, especially by people like him. The uninjured. To him, I was a statistical aberration. What did he know about it? This was my life. Lucky? Right.

He tested my sense of touch. The point of the pin felt sharper on the skin of my left arm and leg than it had last week.

On my right side, I correctly identified sharp or dull and felt the coolness of his fingers when he grasped my right foot.

"Tell me if your foot is up or down?"

I strained to connect my brain to my right foot. Searching for a signal, like a blip on a radar screen, but...nothing. "I don't know. Maybe up? But I'm guessing."

"And now?"

Again...nothing. "I don't know." My proprioception hadn't improved. So eerie to have no sense of where the right side of my body was positioned in space. As if my arm and leg were free floating, not connected to me at all. A capacity I hadn't even known about before. That had allowed me to walk and run without looking down at my feet, to make sure they were aligned, to make sure they were there. Now, unless my arms and legs were in my sight, I had only this sense of absence on the right: a vague nothingness in place of limbs.

"I'll roll you on one side now." He pulled on latex gloves. "For the digital rectal exam. Then I'm done."

"What?"

"The digital rectal exam. To see whether your injury is complete or incomplete."

"No one has done that to me since I was in the emergency room. Dr. Davis explained to me how it's used. You don't need to do it. I'm obviously incomplete. My arm and legs move."

"But it's on the form."

"I don't care."

"It'll only take a few seconds."

"That's not the point. The exam is over. *Now.*"

"You don't have to be so nasty." He gathered his notes and materials and huffed out of my room.

After he left, tears rolled down the sides of my cheeks, wetting my ears.

Clumsily, I wiped my face with my left hand.

Stop. I had to stop. I hadn't cried since the accident. I wouldn't start now. Especially not because of him!

Several nurses had commented on my lack of tears. Shock, they said, but I knew it wasn't. As a child, my father had called me a suck when I cried. Told me I was needy, manipulative, a martyr, like my mother. I didn't know what a martyr was, but I knew it was bad, something I didn't want to be.

The only time I'd cried, really cried, was in the months after Daniel and I had separated. I was overcome by waves of sobs, unpredictable and inconvenient, on the bus to work, on the treadmill at the gym, in the book stacks at the library. A sharp ache, an exposed nerve, raw and throbbing. Endless weeping, like my heart had been ripped from me.

Then finally, I stopped. I simply stopped. I had hardened myself again. I was invulnerable, untouchable. No one, nothing was going to hurt me.

Especially not Dr. Pinkus with his clumsy arrogance, his prodding and poking. This was my home for now. My room was my sanctuary. This was my holiday weekend too. I wasn't a specimen, the final part of an assignment. He had no right to treat me like that. I'd report him to Dr. Davis on Tuesday.

■ ■ ■

Saturday morning. Outside, the sun shimmered in a clear open sky. I glimpsed the trio of walkers crossing the path under my window. Early for them, maybe the holiday had altered their routine too. They wore cotton knit sweaters, the man in baby blue, the women in pink. Must be a warm day because they always dressed sensibly. Maybe after lunch Lisa and I could take a walk on the wooded trail behind the hospital.

My attention drifted to the bedside table, to the autumn leaves and pinecones my mom and I had collected a few days ago. Since the injury, my intact senses seemed heightened, more acute than before, and experiencing these familiar objects had been an unexpected pleasure: inhaling the sharp pine resin, the loamy leaves; the bumpy scales of the cone, the smooth skin of the leaves when I'd brushed them against my cheek.

Last night I'd been completely drained by the encounter with Dr. Pinkus, but this morning I felt strong and energized. When was Lisa going to get here?

In the empty space of waiting, my eyes darted to the drawer of the nightstand. The letter. Not far from my mind since I'd received it two days ago; maybe with Lisa beside me, I'd be ready to read it.

I slid the drawer open and stared at the envelope. My mother hadn't said anything when she'd handed me the card but hadn't offered to open it either, as she did with all my other mail. A tacit acknowledgment. She knew. But I knew that she knew. Her silence had been bridged once about ten years ago in a drunken tirade when I was home from university for a visit.

"You remember Mr. Semple, your old science teacher? Well, my friend Patricia teaches with him. Everyone suspects he's seduced one of his students. And that it's happened before. Even at *other* schools," my mother said. "If you know anything, you should report it." She stared at me bleary-eyed. "You owe it...it's a moral obligation...to protect other girls."

"I don't know what you're talking about." I left the room to pack and catch the next train to Toronto. Twelve-year-old Kathryn clung to me and sobbed, "Don't go. Please don't go." Unbearable, gently peeling her small hands from around my waist, but I had to leave, distance was my only way to survive.

I took out the envelope, turned it in my hand. In the upper left-hand corner, a name I hadn't thought about in years. How had he found out about my accident? To reach me? Maybe through my mother's friend? Maybe someone else? This injury was like a beacon, not only were my parents thrust back into my life, but would I be forced to revisit every relationship? Compelled to remember things long put away and best forgotten?

Mr. Semple would probably be arrested now, but in the early 1980s the teachers and administrators had just turned their heads and he'd been transferred to another high school the following year. Nobody had ever questioned me. Nothing was ever said.

At the time, I'd considered it an affair. An adventure enlivening my dreary days at school where I'd wandered through the gray halls feeling like the walls were closing in. My limbs were so heavy they'd felt like weighted sandbags as I'd dragged myself from class to class. But with Mr. Semple, something had *finally* been happening to me, like a character in a novel.

Though as a hero, he'd hardly cut a dashing figure: short, pale, and dumpy, slicked back hair, reeking of hair lotion, dressed in polyester leisure suits and pleather loafers, he'd picked me up for trysts in the back of his family's two-toned station wagon.

Revolting to think of. Ludicrous. A pathetic cliché. What did he want from me now? I tucked the envelope back in the drawer.

"Hello!" Lisa burst into the room.

Wearing jeans and a black sweater, a fawn leather belt slung low over her hips, her hair shiny and clean, just a touch of lipstick, she was beautiful. Would I ever be pretty again?

"It's great to see you." She attempted a hug, but seated in the chair, framed by the metal halo, I was difficult to touch. "Is this a new wheelchair?"

"I got it yesterday. It's manual. I've graduated from the power chair!" I grinned. "I use my left leg and I can actually move myself! Watch this." Kicking my left leg forward, striking the ground, I pushed off with my foot to propel across the room. My right leg remained on the footrest. "I think the treadmill training is really helping. I'm not walking, but I'm getting closer."

"And no tray on the wheelchair anymore?"

"I haven't needed it for a little while. I feel so much freer without it."

"That's fantastic!" Lisa perched on the bed and opened a bag. "These are from Adam." She handed me two CDs.

"Steven Wright."

"He didn't know what to get, but he wanted to send something."

"Comedy is good."

"And I found this." She held up a book by E.E. Cummings.

"It has the poem we were trying to remember last time I was here. 'Somewhere I have never traveled, gladly beyond.'" As she flipped the pages, something on her hand glinted.

"Is that a ring?"

"Yes." She beamed. "I was just about to tell you. Adam proposed on my birthday. What do you think?"

I hoped my surprise didn't show. They'd been on-again, off-again for years. "It's wonderful. I mean, if it's what you want."

"It is."

"I'm really happy for you. Have you set a date?"

"Next year. Probably late May. We have to finalize arrangements. Will you be my maid of honor?"

No. I wanted to say no. I imagined myself going up the aisle, wheeling my chair with my feet, or if I was lucky, hobbling with a cane, on display, in front of everyone. And what would I wear? What about my hair? My makeup? Would someone have to dress me? If only I could just say no.

But I couldn't. I still had to be a best friend. "Sure…but I don't know what kind of shape I'll be in. I doubt I'll be able to do much to help out, like arranging showers or anything."

"I don't care," Lisa said, taking my hand. "I just want you to be there with me."

"Okay, then. I'll do it." My right leg quivered with a spasm. I placed my left foot on top of my right foot and pushed down gently against it to stop the tremor. "Should we go over to the hospital cafeteria to celebrate? Maybe get some rice pudding? Remember how good it was?" Not the most exciting way to commemorate the occasion, but the best I could think of.

When Lisa went to the washroom, I glanced at the drawer of the nightstand. The letter would have to wait.

■ ■ ■

Later that afternoon, wandering through the forested path behind the hospital, Lisa halted abruptly and pointed. "Look. On that little hill. It's a red fox!"

By the time I spun my wheelchair around, the fox had fled. "I guess I missed it. But that's okay. I'm not really into wildlife these days."

"I can't believe you said that." She laughed. "I guess your sense of humor is returning. You're so strong, you know?"

"Strong? I'm not sure about strong. It's more like I endure. I endure and look forward. Or that's what I'm trying to do."

We continued on. My progress was slow and staggered, and occasionally Lisa pushed me so I could rest my leg. Birds sang, shrill trills and guttural stuttering caws. Squirrels darted through trees, rustling the remaining leaves. The air was fresh, fragrant with the hint of evergreens and moist soil. Scarlet sumac bushes edged the trail, and a few black-eyed Susans and blue cornflowers that had outlasted the frost drooped from their stalks.

"Your mom said she'll come by later and we'll get takeout for dinner. Anything you'd like?" Lisa was staying with my mother at my apartment for the weekend. Strange to think of the two of them there without me.

"I'd love Indian." But Indian food was spicy. Spicy food could stimulate my bowels, possibly resulting in a humiliating accident. Everything had to be so well planned, no room for spontaneity. Even the few choices I had left were constrained by my injury. "Maybe I'd rather have Greek," I pretended. "I know a good place. My mom can pick it up on the way."

"Your mom seems to be coping with everything pretty well," Lisa said.

"She's been great. There's a lot to deal with—the insurance company, government forms—she's doing everything. I'll have to take over eventually, but for now I can just concentrate on getting better."

"How long has it been since she stopped drinking?"

"Five years. Maybe almost six."

"She told me last night that she sees this as a way to make things up to you."

"She kind of said the same thing to me. That she was grateful to AA because they had helped her to be here for me." A confession of sorts, an admission of how she'd treated me in the past. "But I don't know…. It's probably unfair, but it bothered me. That somehow my accident could be a kind of opportunity." I bristled when I thought about it. This was my tragedy. My broken life. My devastation should not be a way to make amends. Not even for my mother.

"We turn here to the left," I said when the path forked. "If we go right, it just leads to the parking lot. This way loops back through the woods to the rehab center."

Lisa pointed to some scrubby bushes at the trunk of an old maple. "There are some purple flowers over by that tree. I'm going to pick some for your room."

As she walked toward the wildflowers, I thought more about my mother. How much she supported me. I'd be lost without her. I knew that. But I hated this forced return to dependence. This new closeness between us was uncomfortable. Sometimes, it rubbed like sandpaper. I wavered from gratitude to resentment to guilt. Was I the problem? Could I not forgive her? Was that it?

A few minutes later, we arrived at the end of the path, a few feet from the hospital entrance.

"Do you want to sit for a while?" Lisa said. "It's so nice out."

We headed to the gardens, still fully lit by the afternoon sun. I parked beside a bench. Lisa moved to help me apply the brakes on my wheelchair. "It's okay," I said. "They put extensions on the brakes so I can reach them myself." I leaned down a little and locked the brake on the left side. "The right side is harder, but I can do it now too!" I crossed my left arm over my lap and bent down, contracting my abdominal muscles for stability the way Barb had instructed yesterday. "See?"

"You are getting so much better." Lisa sat on the bench. "Have you thought about what you're going to do? When this is over and you're out of here?"

"Not really."

"What about your men?"

"My men?" I laughed. "I don't quite think of them that way. Things are pretty much over with Gary. He still visits, helps with my stretches, comes to physio sometimes, cheers me on. We're still friends. But since I told him I don't want to live with him, he's been awkward and distant."

"What about Daniel?"

"I'll probably always love him, but it's too difficult. I can't really see us getting back together. I wish I could, but…."

"So, what will you do? You don't want to go back to your research job, do you?"

"Definitely not." I cringed. "I was so unhappy, but…." I'd stayed. For almost two years, I'd stayed.

I continued to believe that my accident was random and not the result of fate or karma. I knew not even Gary was to blame. Sometimes terrible things just happened, and this had happened to me. But occasionally, late at night, doubt crept in. Maybe there *was* a reason. Maybe I was being punished for wasting my life, for my lack of direction, for my inability to act. Maybe that's why this had happened. To force me to wake up. To start living my life as if I mattered.

Over the summer, I *had* started to think about moving forward, changing my life. At least I'd done that.

"You know, just before this happened I was considering moving back to Toronto. Going back to school. Finishing my doctorate. I wrote a draft of my dissertation proposal in August."

"That's what you should do."

"Even if I'm in a wheelchair, I'd be okay at York. It's accessible and they have resources for students with disabilities." I'd liked that about the university when I'd been a full-time graduate student. There were students with white canes, with working dogs, students using wheelchairs, and other mobility devices. Anybody could go there; everyone was included. Odd to think that now, I was one of the ones to be included. But if other people with disabilities could do it, I could too. "That's what I'm going to do. For sure."

"You know I'll help with anything you need." Lisa stood up and stretched. "I'm going in to get a coffee. Do you want to come?"

"I'll stay here."

"Want anything?"

"No. Thanks." My left arm and hand were much better, but I still couldn't bring a cup to my mouth without spilling the liquid. I needed my long straw, and it was in my room. Annoying. But I didn't really want a coffee anyway.

Toronto. I'd move back to Toronto. Go back to school. A plan. A goal. Something to strive toward. To look forward to. In a year or two, I could be a psychology intern like Angela, the woman from my statistics class I'd seen in the halls almost a month ago. I imagined counseling others, maybe those like me with physical injuries who needed to rebuild their lives. Even like this, I could still finish my PhD. Even like this, I could reclaim that part of myself. Lisa's question had been a gift, giving me a future. And even if I was still using a wheelchair in May, I could be her maid of honor too. My life had been interrupted. My life had been drastically altered. But it wasn't over.

OCTOBER 13

"ARE YOU GOING to the party in the Laurentians tonight?"
I asked as Martha dressed me. "The other nurses have been
talking about it all week."

"That's more for the younger girls." Martha placed my
right foot through the leg of my shorts. "Do you want to try
your left leg?"

From where I was lying on my back on the bed, I bent
my left knee and wiggled my foot through the opening in the
shorts. Then I lifted my bum a few inches up into a bridge
and she slid the shorts over my hips.

I now helped with the morning routine: fed myself breakfast, brushed my teeth with an electric toothbrush, and raised
my left arm to make it easier for Martha as she slipped on my
T-shirt and adjusted it over the halo vest. But my right arm
remained stubbornly flaccid.

"Martha? If just my left arm gets better, will I be able to
dress myself? I mean, can people dress themselves with just
one arm?"

"Of course they can. People who've had strokes do it all
the time. And you're doing well. Really well. Now where have

your socks gone to?" She rummaged through the drawer of the nightstand.

"My mom did the laundry yesterday. She might've put them in the cupboard."

"Here we go." Martha returned with a pair of socks.

"My mom wanted to get everything organized before she went away. She had to go back to London today to sign some papers, extending her leave of absence from work. She'll be back on Sunday."

"So, you're on your own this weekend?"

"I'm supposed to go to Gary's tomorrow for dinner. It's all arranged. The ride with the accessible transit bus there and back. His condo's pretty accessible. Wide enough doorways, an elevator, and no stairs. But I'm kind of nervous. I haven't left the hospital before."

"It'll be good for you to get out."

"That's what Dr. Davis said. I think I'm ready. What are you doing this weekend?"

"Me?" She smiled shyly. "Not much. Saturday, I'll do errands. Probably read some."

"You like to read? Me too. What kind of books do you like?"

"Mostly romances. Like Danielle Steel. I can read for hours. I love getting lost in them."

"I miss reading. Even though I can turn the page now with my left arm, my concentration is terrible. I just can't focus on a whole page. The doctors say it's shock. I hope they're right and it's not some kind of brain damage."

"They'd tell you if it was. Don't worry. Your concentration will come back. You've been through a lot."

"I've started reading poetry, short passages, and articles. That seems to be okay."

"You have to give yourself time."

"I know. But it's hard." I had to be so patient with everything else. Why couldn't the supposedly intact part of me work like it used to? Why couldn't I at least have that? "So, what else will you do this weekend?"

"Well, on Sunday I'll go to church with my dad and my daughter. My dad drives us. He's such a sweet man. So good to me. Then after the service, we always go to one of those Chinese buffet places for brunch. It's my favorite day."

"Sounds nice. Your husband doesn't go?"

"Him?" She chuckled. "Oh no. He just likes to stay home and watch TV. He doesn't like going out at all. That's why I'm so lucky to have my father and daughter. They're great company. Though my daughter gets frustrated with my husband."

"How come?"

"Like last year. It was our twenty-fifth wedding anniversary. And my daughter, she's got a part-time job while she goes to college, so she saved up and bought us a gift certificate to a really nice steak place. But we couldn't get Stan, my husband, to go. He kept saying next weekend, we'll go then. So, the day before the certificate expired, my daughter and I ended up going. She was some mad at her father."

"Were you upset?"

"Not really. She and I had a real nice meal. And I wasn't that surprised. As I said, my husband doesn't like to leave the house." Martha picked up the brush. "Do you want me to braid your hair?"

"If you don't mind. It keeps it away from my face."

"Your hair's getting long, way past your shoulders, nearly to the middle of your back." She twisted an elastic band on the end of the plait. "I'll be back a little later to transfer you to your chair."

After she left, I pictured Martha and her daughter celebrating her wedding anniversary in the restaurant, then imagined Martha curled in a chair, devouring romance novels while her husband lay sprawled on a couch, a remote in his hand in the blue light of a television screen. Kind of sad. And yet she didn't seem particularly unhappy; in fact, in her own quiet way, she seemed relatively content. Maybe it had to do with expectations. Settling for less.

Not me. I'd always wanted more. When I'd felt stuck as a teenager in London, and more recently here, after my separation, I'd known deep down that eventually I'd be able to improve things, to create a better life. Even now, the future motivated me: seeing myself walking, resuming my independence, and finishing my doctorate. Once again, I'd leave a terrible situation behind. I was good at this. I knew what to do.

But this time was different. Before, I could always will myself to act. No matter how frightened or sad, I never doubted that I was in charge of my fate. But now, no matter how hard I pushed, no matter how hard I tried, I couldn't completely influence the extent of my recovery. My body's ultimate limits were beyond my control, and I couldn't escape the final outcome. This time, reinventing myself would be harder. This time, I might have to settle for less.

■ ■ ■

Later that evening, a few minutes before eleven, Amy, one of the regular night nurses, popped into my room. "Do you need anything else before I finish my shift?"

"If you could turn out the lights, that'd be great. I'm ready to sleep."

"No problem." She fluffed the pillows around my head. "Just ten more minutes, then I'm heading to the mountains!"

"You're driving up to the party tonight?"

"I'm off the rest of the weekend. We've booked the cabin until Sunday, so I want to get the most out of it. The car's packed and I'm all set to go." Amy grinned. "I'm bringing the fixings for shooters. Though everyone will probably be loaded by the time I get there. It's always a blast. The rehab party retreat. We do it every year."

"I hope you have a good time."

"Thanks." She flipped the light switch. "I'll see you next week."

I closed my eyes to sleep, but I was jittery and tense. I hadn't felt that way before Amy had come in, with the reminder that for others, life happened outside these walls: drinking, partying, having fun. Or maybe something about Amy's excitement, her carefree attitude, had bothered me. Despite a two-hour drive on pitch black, winding mountain roads, Amy assumed she'd arrive unharmed.

And she would. And all the other nurses would, too. They could travel at night, their lives not ruined or destroyed by a simple road trip. They'd be fine. Not like me. Because of a road trip, I'd never be fine again.

It was so unfair. Not that I wanted them to be hurt. I didn't. It wasn't their fault. But it hadn't been my fault either. "It came out of nowhere. There was nothing I could do," Gary said. But he hadn't been hurt. A few scratches and bruises. Only me. A moose. A fucking moose on a four-lane highway!

The emergency room doctor from Hawkesbury, the one who had saved my life, had called a few days after the accident, when I was still in the neuro-observation unit. My mom had held the phone to my ear so we could talk, though I'd been so disoriented, I'd barely processed her words.

I remembered them now. Five fatalities due to moose collisions along the same stretch of highway that summer and only I had survived. "Someone must've been watching out for you that night," the doctor had said. "You're a very lucky girl."

There was that word again. *Lucky!* It was so easy for others to say. But if there was a God who had been looking out for me, why had the accident occurred at all? Why hadn't he spared me? Just left me alone?

And that horrible Dr. Pinkus, citing the statistics, my good fortune at defying the odds. But if the odds were really in my favor, the accident shouldn't have happened at all, or at least I should have been able to walk away, like Gary.

Instead, something terrible had happened. Something terrible had happened to me! My right arm quivered, then tremored more violently. That was it. That was all my right arm could do. Shake with a spasm. So little of me worked and might never work again. It was so unfair.

The stories of other patients didn't help. Most of them had themselves to blame—they had been drunk or high behind the wheel of cars, motorcycles, ATVs—but I had done nothing wrong. I felt targeted. My life was ruined, and it wasn't even my fault. Targeted. Alone and targeted.

A couple of days ago, in the pages of the *Ottawa Citizen*, I'd been drawn to the Local News section listing the car accidents, injuries, and fatalities.

"Anything interesting?" my mother had asked, peering up from her book.

"No." I didn't want her to know what had captured my attention. I scanned the headlines: "Manotick-area man loses hand in motorcycle collision;" "Hwy 417 reopens after three-vehicle crash;" and "Man suffers life-threatening injuries in rollover."

I read every word. A van from the oncoming lane had flipped and landed on the man's car. A crushed roof trapped him behind the wheel until emergency workers cut him free. The driver of the van had escaped injury. Like Gary. But the car driver was critically injured. Still in Intensive Care. An innocent victim, seriously damaged. Like me. Finally I'd found someone like me.

News about my accident had appeared in a newspaper too, a local Francophone press near Hawkesbury. Gary's cousin who lived in the area had given him a copy. I'd insisted on seeing it, and he'd finally brought it to me last week. In moments alone, I took it out and stared at it, completely transfixed. It wasn't even an article, just a black and white photo in the middle of a page: a dead moose lying on the shoulder of the highway beside Gary's crumpled, compact car. The caption read: "Une femme, 31, d'Ottawa était sérieusement blessée."

I studied it closely as if by careful scrutiny I could recapture that dreadful moment that had split my life into *before* and *after*, the transition from complete wellness to bodily devastation. As if this picture could fill the void in my memory and allow me to fully understand what had happened, what had gone wrong.

I conjured the grainy photograph in my mind. Imagined the photographer roused from his bed that night to take the shot while I, absent from the frame and barely alive, had been in the back of an ambulance speeding toward a hospital, leaving my former life behind.

The muscles in my chest constricted. My legs trembled. Such an awful thing, such a terrible, terrible thing had happened to me. There was no way back. And the future was so terrifyingly unknown. How would I ever manage my ruined life?

I closed my eyes and took deep, deliberate breaths. I had to get some rest. Force myself forward. I was strong. I could do it. Every day I was a little better. Hopefully, that would continue. And if not, there were ways of learning to be different in the world. Other people—amazing people—had done it. Helen Keller. Stephen Hawking. Peter from work. I could do it too.

Tomorrow, I'd be re-entering the world for the first time since the accident. Dinner at Gary's was another step toward recovery, toward reclaiming a semblance of normalcy, an approximation of a life.

OCTOBER 14

IN THE LOBBY of the rehab center, I angled my chair to face the main entrance, so I'd spot the driver as soon as they arrived. I'd seen the drivers here before, picking up other patients. They'd stride through the sliding doors, announce the name of their pickup, and wait just a few minutes, at most, before posting a "Sorry We Missed You" card on the wall. Today, a driver would be calling my name.

I lowered my eyes. The bus ticket was on my lap under my left hand. My right hand lay limp across my right thigh, covered in scabs from various IV insertion points. I should have asked a nurse to cover it with a bandage.

I checked the clock on the wall. Just ten more minutes before the driver was scheduled to pick me up and take me to Gary's condo.

Ten more minutes. My right leg shook: up and down, up and down. I tried to press it against the wheelchair's footrest to lessen the tremors but, though the right leg was getting stronger, I couldn't muster enough force to quiet it. I moved my left foot on top of the right, pushed gently, and the right leg settled down. There. Relax. It's okay. Just relax.

But fear gnawed at me, increasing with each movement of the clock's minute hand. Was I really ready to go *out there*? Images invaded my mind: crushed metal and shattered glass, the whine of sirens piercing the air. A dark night with flashes of light. A paramedic leaning over me, shouting my name.

"Susan? Susan Mockler?"

I was startled as a burly uniformed man approached me. The driver. Of course. "Right here," I said.

My stomach lurched as the driver pulled out of the parking lot. Trees, sidewalks, cars, and pedestrians blurred by. I closed my eyes to quell the dizziness. My arms and legs jerked with spasms at each bump in the road. After a few minutes, I felt better and looked out the window. Color flooded my vision: the sky, blue and unending, interrupted by splotches of crimson and orange, the last autumn leaves still clinging to branches. Everything seemed bright and shiny and new.

When we crossed the Pretoria Bridge, memory intruded: the paths along the canal where I'd walked, jogged, and biked. The driver turned on to Bank Street. My apartment was less than a block away, but the four steps at the entrance now posed an impossible barrier. So close to home, yet so far away. Here, but not here. Here in a different way.

We continued further south into the Glebe, passing stores and restaurants I'd been in dozens of times, but I felt disconnected. I didn't belong.

"Left or right here, Miss?"

"What?"

"Do I turn left or right at the next intersection?"

I glanced out the window. Where were we? Near Carleton? The Experimental Farm? I was disoriented. "I'm not sure."

"You don't know where you're going?"

"I do, but...."

"Where do I turn?"

"I'm going to a friend's place. I can't remember exactly where he lives." I took a deep breath. "I haven't left the hospital in over two months. I gave them the address when I called. Don't you know how to find it?"

"I will." The driver paged through a street atlas. "Don't you worry, young lady. I'll find it."

But why couldn't I remember? I'd driven there countless times. Despite what the doctors said, I still worried about brain damage. Reaching into my memory, where I expected details, there were these gaps. Mostly for events in the time just before the accident. A confusion, a buzzing blankness like static, that I could no longer bring into focus. Mild retrograde amnesia from the concussion was possible, the doctors had said, but more likely shock. Shock. Could this really only be shock? Would it ever go away? Were they right? Was I cognitively intact? In moments like this, I tried to believe them, tried not to panic, tried to believe that my brain was okay. My brain was okay, and I was okay.

"Here we are." The driver pulled up to Gary's condominium. He unbuckled my seatbelt, unhooked the straps tethering my wheelchair to the floor, and then released the brakes on the chair. "You're good to go. Do you want me to take you in?"

"No." I wheeled down the bus's ramp.

"Good luck to you."

On the sidewalk, I used my left leg to pivot my chair toward the entrance. No one was around, and I paused for a moment. A gray squirrel scurried across the lawn, a gentle breeze stirred the leaves on the trees and caressed my cheeks. Despite the warmth of the October day, I detected the crisp, smoky scent of autumn in the air. I loved this time of year and here I was enjoying it, away from the hospital, outside, on my own.

In my peripheral vision, through the bars of the halo, I saw Gary. He strolled down the walkway, waving as he approached, dressed in a colorful array of sports paraphernalia, clothes that I recognized even from a distance. A royal blue cap sat backward on his head, an attempt to conceal his increasing baldness, and a red and black hockey jersey topped his teal soccer shorts. The overall effect was not unlike a children's cartoon character.

I smiled as he came nearer. I was looking forward to the rest of the day.

In his condo a few minutes later, Gary said, "My mom and my daughter are joining us for dinner."

"*What?*" My hand shook, splashing water as I placed the plastic tumbler on the kitchen table. "I don't want anyone to see me like this."

"I thought it would be fun. It's just family."

"They're not my family."

"My mom has been worried about you. She wanted to come. And Crystal's living with me full-time now. I could hardly ask her to stay away."

"She couldn't have had dinner with her mother? Just this one night? Crystal hates me."

"That's not true." Gary turned to stir a pot of sauce on the stove.

But it *was* true. Whenever he had compelled the three of us to be together, to have dinner or watch a video on TV, Crystal had shrugged away any of my overtures, glared at me sullenly, talked only to her father, and pretended I didn't exist.

Most of the time, I didn't want to be there either. But I had nowhere else to go. It had been easy to fall in with Gary after Daniel left. We had fun: cycled, hiked, skated, and skied. As long as we didn't talk too much, I was okay. I suspected Crystal blamed me for her parents' divorce. But if Gary had thought he was leaving his wife for me, I'd never encouraged it, hadn't promised him anything. I refused to feel responsible. I was struggling enough in my own life.

"When are they coming?" I asked when Gary joined me at the table.

"Around five."

"What time is it now?"

"About four-thirty."

"If you'd told me about this, I never would have come. My pickup's not until six-thirty. I can't believe you did this to me."

"It'll be fine."

"What are you making for dinner?"

"Spaghetti and meatballs."

"I can't eat that. It's too difficult. I can only eat with my adapted spoon."

"I thought it would be a nice change from hospital food. I'm going to cut yours up and put it in a bowl."

"I'm not eating that way in front of them. Like an infant."

"They'll understand."

"I don't want to be seen like that."

"I could make you a cheese sandwich. Would that be better?"

"Make sure you cut it in quarters *before* you bring it to the table. After that, I can manage on my own."

Gary bustled around: setting the table, folding napkins, and laying out placemats. He hummed "Hotel California" as he retrieved glasses and plates from cupboards; knives, forks, and spoons from drawers; adjusting and readjusting each setting until everything was lined up, everything was in order.

"There." He stepped back. "Doesn't that look pretty?"

"Why did you have to invite them here tonight?"

"Maybe I should add some candles." He surveyed the table. "That'd be nice." He poked through a drawer. "Where are those tea lights?"

"Gary! Stop it. Answer me."

"I told you," he said, still searching the drawer. "I thought—"

"*What?* What did you think?"

"That they'd want to see you. That…."

"It's my first time out of the hospital and I'm still in the halo. You should have known that I wouldn't want other people here."

"I guess I thought that it'd be easier. That you didn't want to spend time alone with me anymore."

"What are you talking about?"

He faced me gripping a plastic bag of tea lights. "I think you know."

"Because I don't want to move in with you after I'm out of rehab?"

"That's part of it."

"I can't commit to anything but myself right now."

"I don't know where that leaves me. Especially now that you're planning to move back to Toronto. I really don't see where this leaves me at all."

"Not this again. I thought you were my friend."

"I am. But—"

The intercom rang. My body jolted in response.

"She's early." He pressed the entry key to unlock the lobby door. "Come on in, Mom. I'll meet you at the elevator."

A few minutes later, I heard footsteps and voices coming down the hall and caught myself readying my face with a smile. So automatic, I'd almost been unaware of it, years of practice, of forced grins and false reassurances. Everything's okay, everything's fine.

But it wasn't. Not today.

"Where's Susan?" Gary's mother asked as they entered the condo.

"Right in the kitchen, Mom. She's been looking forward to your visit."

"Hi, Edna," I said.

Her jaw slackened; her eyes brightened with alarm. "Goodness. I didn't realize that *thing* was screwed right into your head." She indicated the halo with a fluttering hand. "But it's good to see you, dear." Taking a seat at the table, she reached out tentatively and patted my arm. "And you *are* looking well."

I almost laughed out loud. Compared to what? A *corpse*?

"I baked some ginger cookies for you to take home." She set a plastic container on the table.

Home? A funny word to use. Where was my home? "Thank you. That's very kind."

"I remembered you liked them and...well...I'm so sorry I haven't been to see you. I just can't go to the hospital. Too many bad memories of when I had my mastectomy. I hope you understand, dear."

"Of course."

"But Gary's been keeping me up to date, haven't you?"

"Sure have," he said. "Can I get you a drink, Mom? I have cranberry juice and sparkling water."

"Water is fine for me."

"Do you want anything else, Susan?"

"No." I'd spilled water just setting the tumbler on the table a few minutes ago and I still sometimes dribbled liquid on my shirt when I drank from a cup. I didn't need anyone to witness *that*.

Gary brought the water to his mother and then moved to the counter, chopping vegetables for the salad. "Let's see... cucumbers, radishes, maybe some tomato?"

"Daddy...I'm home." Crystal swept into the room, infusing the air with a vanilla scent. "Oh." She stopped abruptly when she saw her grandmother and me at the table.

"Remember I told you Susan and Granny were going to be here tonight?" Gary said.

"I forgot." She dumped her shopping bags in a corner. "Hi, Granny." She pecked her cheek. Crystal was wearing khaki cargo pants and a white jean jacket and as she wiggled behind her grandmother's chair, her coat shifted to reveal a black crop top and a silver navel ring. That was new.

171

She flopped down in the seat across from me. "My dad says you're getting better."

"I am. But it takes a long time."

"What's this?" Crystal grabbed the plastic container and pried off the lid. "Cookies!"

"I made those for Susan," Edna said.

"Go ahead," I said. "There's lots."

She grabbed a couple and looked at me again. "Does that thing on your head hurt?"

"No. Even when they were drilling holes in my skull to attach it, it didn't really hurt."

"They drilled holes right in your head? *Gross!*" She bit into a cookie. "Are you in the wheelchair all the time?"

"For now."

"Hey, Dad, remember when we visited Granny in the hospital and how when she was sleeping, you'd take me for rides in her wheelchair, running *really, really* fast, pushing me down the hall?"

"You shouldn't have done that, Gary." Edna clicked her tongue. "I'm surprised the nurses didn't stop you or even ask you to leave."

"It was only once or twice," he said. "When no one else was around."

"It was fun," Crystal said.

"Well, it's not very fun if you *have* to be in a wheelchair," I said. "It's not fun at all."

"Dinner's ready," Gary said. "Crystal, can you help me serve?"

As we settled down to the meal, Crystal blathered on about the things she'd seen at the mall and wanted to buy.

"*Ooh*…and I tried on the most amazing jacket. It's so cute and it's only sixty dollars, but I ran out of money. I absolutely *love* it. Can we go buy it tomorrow, Daddy?"

Was Crystal as vacuous as she seemed? *Beverly Hills, 90210* was her favorite show, and she thought Tori Spelling had the perfect life. "Her dad's rich, she gets to be a famous TV actress, and live in LA. I'm *soooo* jealous. But I'm prettier, right, Daddy?"

At fifteen, I had been so different. Obsessed with literature and music, filling notebooks with angst-ridden poetry about death and decay. Trying to read Sartre and Kierkegaard and other philosophers I didn't understand. A different kind of stereotype, a little like Ally Sheedy in *The Breakfast Club*, but even now, I still thought it was a better one.

Edna ate slowly, deliberately, cutting her spaghetti with a knife and fork, saving her salad for last. Gary and Crystal swirled strands of pasta onto spoons with their forks and alternated bites of salad and spaghetti. Forks and knives, forks and spoons, the synchronous use of cutlery, the simplicity of eating. I didn't even attempt to reach down and grasp a quarter of my sandwich. I refused to expose the challenge that feeding myself still posed. Sometimes my left arm quavered, and my coordination was awkward and imprecise. Besides, if I'd been hungry when I'd arrived, my appetite had vanished. I'd eat a sandwich later. At the rehab center. Alone. In my room.

"There's an old-timers' soccer game tomorrow afternoon," Gary said. "Want to come along, Crystal? Watch your old man kick the ball around?"

"Can we go to the Rideau Centre first and get that jacket? *Please?*"

"Sure, honey. I have to get some new cleats before the game. You can help me pick them out."

"That's *so* terrible you lost your old pair in the accident."

The word *accident* alerted me, and I listened carefully.

"They towed the car before I had a chance to get my stuff," Gary said. "But on the bright side, the insurance company is giving me money to buy some new ones."

"But it's still so awful. They were your favorites, weren't they?" Crystal said.

"I can't believe you are talking about *fucking* soccer shoes!" My legs started to tremor. "I lost the ability to *move* in that accident."

"Come on, Susan," Gary said. "It's completely different. You know we didn't mean it like that."

I backed away from the table. Crystal smirked. Edna stared down at her plate and fiddled with her fork. My legs now shook vigorously with spasms. I hated this. How I could no longer hide my feelings. Another way my body betrayed me. Something else I could no longer control. I tried to keep my voice steady. "I'm going home now. I mean, back to the rehab center."

"You can't do that," Gary said. "Your ride's not going to be here for almost an hour."

"I'll call and see if they'll come earlier."

"You don't have to do this," he said. "You're making a big deal out of nothing."

"Get me the phone." He handed it to me, and I almost choked in frustration. I'd forgotten he had an old phone, with a rotary dial embedded in the handset. I couldn't possibly work this with one hand. At the hospital, I used a speakerphone with large push buttons. So, there could be no dramatic exit, no storming from the room, no slamming of doors. Even escaping this horrible situation required Gary's help. "Can you get the card out of my bag? It's got their number on it. I'll need you to dial it for me."

"Are you sure you want to leave now?"

"Yes."

I held the receiver to my ear, my left hand trembled from its weight, but I was determined to make the call on my own.

"They can come earlier. They'll be here in ten minutes." I passed Gary the telephone to hang up. "Can you take me downstairs? I'll wait out front."

In the lobby, I asked Gary to open the door of the main entrance. "I'd prefer to be outside."

"You don't want me to stay with you?"

"No. But I want you to look at me. *Really* look at me. *This* is what happened to *me* in the accident. How could you even talk about your soccer shoes when I was right there? Why didn't you stop Crystal?"

"I told you, it's different. And when I look at you, I see how you were before and how you'll be again."

"But this is how I am now. And I may not get better." My voice caught in my throat, a rush of sadness that surprised me.

"I like to stay positive. I know you're going to recover." He moved closer and reached out his arm.

"Don't touch me. Leave me alone."

A few minutes later, I heard footsteps approaching me from behind.

"I brought you these." Edna placed the cookies on my

lap. "I thought you might want them later. You didn't eat any supper."

"Thanks."

"I'm so sorry about what happened. He really spoils her. Always has. And neither of them ever taught her manners or basic consideration for others."

"I think there are things about Crystal and about everything else that Gary just doesn't want to see."

"Do you want some company until your ride comes?"

"I'd like to be alone, but thanks for asking. And for the cookies."

"Not at all. Take care of yourself, dear."

The wind was cooler now against my face, and as the sun descended, bands of pink and purple streaked the sky. More people were out on the street than earlier this afternoon, jogging, pushing strollers, and walking dogs. From time to time, various passersby glanced at me, while others lingered longer with frank stares of curiosity. But I didn't care.

Had Gary always been so insensitive? I'd often been bored with him, but always thought he was decent, basically good. Had I completely misjudged him? Had I been in that much of a fog over the past year and a half?

He'd never apologized to me about the accident. Not once. And while I'd accepted what I'd been told, that there was nothing he could have done, shouldn't he at least say he was sorry for what had happened to me?

Had he changed since the accident, or had I? It was unnerving. As if I'd been gazing at a holographic image that had suddenly sharpened into focus, revealing something unexpected, something almost cruel.

The accessible bus rounded the corner. I thrust my left foot forward, pushed off the pavement, and wheeled down the sidewalk. I was so relieved to be getting away from here and returning to a place I belonged.

OCTOBER 20

"WHERE IS YOUR moisturizer?" my mom asked. "Do you think Martha might have put it in your cupboard?"

"You can check," I said.

My mom opened the cabinet and rummaged through one of the drawers. "Look what I found." She held up a small, brown glass bottle.

"It's the holy water from Lourdes that Dad brought. A lady from the Legion gave it to him. Remember?"

"What should I do with it?"

"Why don't we try putting some on my bladder? It can't hurt. And I really, really want to be able to pee again." I worried about needing catheters for the rest of my life. My left arm was promising, I was pretty sure it would continue to strengthen and be restored. But the right arm wasn't really improving. I might not get it back. With only my left hand working, I'd be unable to catheterize myself. And without bladder function, I'd require an attendant. I'd never be independent again.

Before my accident, when I'd seen someone in a wheelchair, I thought they just couldn't walk. I'd had no idea what else could be involved. How, with a spinal cord injury, all of your systems shut down. How arms were more important than legs. How not being able to walk was just a small part of it.

My mom lifted my T-shirt.

"I think your bladder is somewhere around here?"

"I think so too. I'm sure it's close enough."

She unstoppered the bottle and dabbed some of the holy water on my lower abdomen.

"It's worth a try," she said, smiling.

I giggled. "Why not?" I didn't really believe anything would happen, but since my injury, I was willing to find hope anywhere.

■ ■ ■

The next afternoon after lunch we were sitting outside.

"Soon, it will be too cold for this," my mom said. "Should we go for a walk along the path?"

"Maybe in a bit." I was enjoying the sun on my face. The crispness of the air. I didn't really want to move. I became aware of a familiar pressure, almost a tingling in my lower abdomen. The feeling grew stronger, more intense. "I think I'm going to pee!"

"Really?" My mom looked surprised.

"What should I do?" I asked. "Should I just pee in the chair? I'm afraid if I try to hold it, I might lose the urge."

"Just go ahead," my mom said.

"But I'll make a mess."

"The nurses won't mind cleaning you up. They'll understand."

And so, I did. I felt a release and a slight wetness on my right side, under my bum.

"It worked! I can pee again!"

That night my mother daubed holy water on my right hand and arm and again on my lower abdomen near where we figured my colon was. This time, though, there were no sudden improvements. Not in my right hand, not in my right arm, and not in my bowels. I'd known that the return of my bladder function had just been a coincidence, that the holy water hadn't really been the cause. But a tiny part of me had wished a small miracle had occurred, and that maybe it would happen again.

OCTOBER 30

SEATED IN MY CHAIR at one end of the parallel bars, I waited for Sheila, my physiotherapist, to return with the video camera. I eyed the bars, keyed up, like I was at the starting line of a race. I felt a whirring, a heightened awareness of my body and what I hoped it would achieve.

Over the past two weeks, the strength and function in both my legs had increased dramatically. Whether it was the treadmill training, the strengthening exercises I did every day in physio, or some combination, I wasn't sure, but it was thrilling. Last week, I'd taken a few tentative steps on my own, my left arm gripping the railing for support, but today Sheila had decided I was ready to walk the full length of the parallel bars. Nine meters. It would have been effortless just a few months ago, but it was a marathon now.

What was taking Sheila so long? And my mom? I'd promised we wouldn't start without her. I knew she'd arrive soon. Unlike the mother of the past, this one could be counted on.

My mom waved to me from the doorway. "I went up to your room first," she said, when she reached the parallel bars. "I didn't think you'd be here already."

"I came down a few minutes ago."

"I brought your water." She held up the thermal cup with the long straw. "How are you feeling?"

"Good. Excited." The thrill of what I was about to do came flooding back. Walk. Today I was going to *walk*. "Here's Sheila now…and Kyle."

"Sorry I took so long," Sheila said. "Couldn't find the camera. Joyce, have you met Kyle? He's the physio assistant on the body-weight support team."

"Sure, we've met," Kyle said. "Susan's mom's been in a few times to watch her on the treadmill."

"Of course," Sheila said.

"More than a few," my mom said, smiling.

"Kyle's going to be our cameraman today. We definitely want to record this for the study. You ready, Susan?"

Sheila crouched, facing me, her arms extended in a spotter's stance. "Joyce, can you get behind Susan, and once she's up, follow with the chair in case she needs to sit down?"

"Sure." My mom positioned herself behind my wheelchair and grabbed the handles. "I'm all right here?"

"Perfect," Sheila said. "Okay, let's give it a try!"

With my left hand, I grasped the bar beside me, leaned forward in my chair, transferred my weight to my feet, and pulled myself to stand. I was up! Ready to go!

"Start with the left," Sheila said.

I swung my left leg and took a step. It moved well, almost normally. I paused and slid my left hand ahead on the bar. I concentrated on my right leg, pushed down on the ball of my foot for leverage, then lifted it in the air. So heavy, as if a fifty-pound weight were attached to my ankle. Thrusting forward, my leg was like steel, refusing to bend at the knee. But still, the foot found its way, winging to the side to clear the floor, and landing just in front of my left foot. Now, another step with the left. And another with the right. Left then right. Left then right. I inched along. Perspiration streamed down my face.

"Do you want to take a break?" Sheila asked.

"No," but I stood for a moment and caught my breath. I scanned the remaining length of the bar. Endless. The bar was endless. I stepped forward with my left and again forced my right leg to step. Step. Step. Left. Right. Step. Step. I was almost two-thirds of the way! My right leg shook with a spasm. I pressed down on the foot, weighting the leg to stop it. Step. Step. Left. Right. Step. Step.

"I made it!" I collapsed into the chair, breathing heavily. "That was hard. Really hard." But I'd done it. I'd really done it!

"I'm so proud of you, honey," my mom said.

"Way to go!" Kyle said.

"Excellent work," Sheila said.

"Can I have some water?"

My mother passed me the jug, her eyes teary. "You were terrific," she said.

■ ■ ■

That night in bed, my nerves and muscles hummed together in an internal reverberation. Walking. I'd actually been walking. One foot after the other, each pressing into the ground, pushing off in turn, suspended in air, and then again, step by step. Walking!

I still had a long way to go. I was exhausted after only nine meters. I needed to be able to walk much further than that. But it was a promising start. Walking. Over ground. Not on the treadmill. Not in a harness. Just holding on to a bar. And from there, maybe someday with a cane? And then... maybe I really was going to be able to walk again, all the time, just like before.

After I'd finished my session, I'd met Jack in the physio room.

"I saw you up there," he'd said. "You looked great!"

"Thanks." Wheeling toward the door, I overheard him talking to Sheila.

"So how come some people get to walk again and...like, other people don't?"

I knew how he felt. Cheated. The way I had when I'd watched the teenaged girl who'd seemed to fully recover in only a week. And seeing me walk would be even more of a shock. When first admitted to rehab, I'd looked worse than anyone else.

But my injury was incomplete so neurons could still fire, even imperfectly, across the spinal cord. Jack's injury was complete. In his case, neurons were shooting into a black hole. Probably only microns of difference distinguished our injuries: the randomness of where and how the damage had occurred. But even with an incomplete injury, how much more I'd recover was still unknown. Would my right arm and leg, my balance, my gait, my level of independence, continue to improve? No one really knew.

The only certainty for me, for Jack, was the aftermath of our injuries—the hollow ache—the longing for the damage to have never happened, the wish to be whole again.

Enough. I had to sleep. It had been a good day. A great day. I had to focus on that.

NOVEMBER 2

"I NEED MORE water." Granules of bird-seed-like psyllium lodged in my teeth and scratched my throat. Martha passed me my water, and I took a big gulp. Every morning I worried that I wouldn't get the two teaspoons down. I'd read the warning on the package: "Taking this product without adequate fluid may cause it to swell and block the throat or esophagus." I always made sure I drank a lot of water when I took it. I'd survived too much to be suffocated by a fiber supplement.

"Here's your breakfast," Martha said, setting the tray on my over-bed table. She opened the carton of milk, poured it over the bran cereal, and stuck my long straw in the prune juice. "All set?"

"I am. Thanks."

"I'll be back in a few minutes."

I scooped some bran twigs into my mouth and sipped a little prune juice. Food as medicine. Yuck. Just a few spoonfuls, a few slurps, and my brown breakfast would be done.

"Finished?" Martha asked, returning to the room.

"Yes."

She pushed aside the table and lowered the head of the

186

bed. I rolled on my side. I heard the snap as she pulled on gloves and then felt the wiggle of her finger in my rectum. Digital stimulation: to stimulate the bowel reflex and promote "evacuation." Every morning we had to go through this. Every single morning.

"I think you should have a glycerin suppository today," Martha said. "It's been almost four days since your last bowel movement."

A crinkling of foil as she opened the suppository and then her finger again as she inserted it.

"I'll leave you for fifteen minutes," she said, placing the call bell beside my left arm. "Ring if you get an urge before then."

I waited and waited. A release of gas. Nothing else. In the last week or so I'd started to feel my bowels contracting before a movement. I hoped it was a sign that one day soon this bowel routine—this retraining—would end. But right now, I felt nothing.

"No urge?" Martha asked, returning to my room.

"Nothing."

The commode whined as Martha rolled it across the room. A high toilet seat on wheels, she helped me transfer onto it. She took me to the bathroom and parked me over the toilet.

"I'll leave you here for a little while and we'll see if anything happens," she said, heading out the door.

I grasped the side armrest with my left hand and rocked gently back and forth, trying to set my bowels in motion. Nothing. I rocked again and clenched my abdominal muscles, bearing down. Nothing. The overhead fluorescent light flickered, bathing the room in a greenish pulsing glow. I was hot. Sweat beaded the middle of my forehead and dampened the hair at the base of my neck. I rocked. I pushed. I strained. Nothing.

I rocked again. Dizzy. Queasy. I tugged the cord to call the nursing station.

"Yes?" A voice spoke through the intercom.

"I'm on the commode. I want off."

"Martha's on break. Can you hang on a few more minutes?"

"No. I want off now."

"I'll send someone down as soon as I can."

My legs dangled, not quite reaching the floor. I was stuck here.

My tongue was gummy in my mouth. My stomach churned. I tasted bile. What would happen if I threw up? I couldn't bend my neck because of the halo. Would I choke? Could I lean forward far enough at my waist without falling off the commode? My right leg tremored. I had to get out of here!

I yanked the cord. *Beep. Beep.* Please answer. Please someone answer.

What if this was autonomic dysreflexia? Constipation could cause it. They'd warned me about it. My blood pressure would skyrocket, and I could have a stroke or a seizure. I could die. My head throbbed. I closed one eye, opened it, then closed the other. Was my vision blurry? I couldn't tell. Help! Please someone help! Both my legs shook. What if I tumbled to the floor? The halo smashing into the toilet. My neck breaking again!

"Susan? You okay?" Martha said, entering the bathroom.

"No. Get me out of here!" I rasped. "I need to lie down. Right now."

Martha transferred me to the bed, and I sat down on the side then lay on my back. She raised the head of the bed. "Drink some water." She held my cup under me.

I took a few sips.

"Are you feeling better?"

"Yes." I took a deep breath. "I thought I was going to die in there."

"Someone should have come sooner. They knew I was on break. I'm sorry you had to go through that. We're short-staffed today."

"I felt so terrible. I hate the commode."

"I know. But you're fine. You're not going to die." She smiled gently. "Here you go." She pressed a cold cloth to my forehead and against each eye. "Better?"

"Yeah. Thanks."

"Just rest for a while and I'll come back later to get you ready for physio."

I closed my eyes. Took more deep breaths. I didn't want to get ready. I didn't want to get dressed. I didn't want to go to physio. I was tired of the fight, tired of trying to get my body to do things it didn't want to do. I'd had enough.

NOVEMBER 14

MARTHA RUSHED INTO the room, her face flushed. "Neurology just called. You have an appointment in Dr. Chamberlain's office at the hospital in an hour. We have to get you ready."

"Is it for the halo?"

"I'm pretty sure." She pushed aside the table with my breakfast tray on it.

"But it's supposed to be next week. November twenty-first." I checked the whiteboard calendar on the wall, the date circled and starred by my mother: "Halo off!"

"Well, they want to see you this morning." Martha opened the drawer of the nightstand. "Darn! I have to get you a hospital gown. Be right back."

Months of anticipation and now, completely unexpectedly, it was happening now. Hopefully, my vertebrae were ready. My right arm trembled with a spasm. I was nervous. I didn't want to go to the appointment alone. I moved my eyes to the clock: nine-thirty. My mom was meeting with the rehab consultant. I had no way of reaching her. I wheeled to the phone. Daniel. Maybe he could come.

"Of course," he said. "I'll cancel my meeting and be right over."

That was the thing about Daniel. He could be counted on.

Martha returned with the blue gown. "Let's get you ready to go."

By the time Daniel arrived, Martha and another nurse had shifted me onto a trolley and cranked up one end so I was in a slightly elevated sitting position, my legs straight out in front of me.

"I'm so glad you could come," I said to Daniel. "We're leaving in a few minutes. The porter's on his way."

Daniel walked beside me as the porter wheeled me through the connecting corridors to the hospital.

"I hope it comes off today. I mean, if it's ready."

"It'll probably be easier for you to move around without it," Daniel said.

"Yeah…it weighs about fifteen pounds. And you know what else? I'll be able to have a shower! An actual shower. I couldn't before, because the vest couldn't get wet." No more bed baths. After almost three months, I'd finally feel clean.

When we reached the neurology department, the receptionist handed the porter a requisition for X-rays. About twenty minutes later, we returned from radiology with the films of my cervical spine.

"You can go in now," the receptionist said. The porter took me into the office. Daniel was at my side.

"Think I'll grab a quick smoke while you're in here," the porter said. "Good luck!"

I hadn't seen them in over two months, but when Dr. Chamberlain and the resident, Dr. Murray, entered the room,

I remembered them well. Especially Dr. Murray. In those early, terrifying days, he was my lifeline: explaining the injury, answering my questions, giving me the results of the daily X-rays that assessed the alignment of the fractures once the halo had been attached.

Dr. Chamberlain nodded to me. Dr. Murray smiled.

"This is Daniel," I said. "Is it all right if he stays?"

"Sure." Dr. Chamberlain shrugged. "Take a seat."

"Thanks." Daniel squeezed my hand and headed to a chair on the far side of the room.

"How have you been?" Head down, Dr. Chamberlain paged through my chart.

"I'm doing well. I can use my left arm and my left leg pretty well. My bladder function has returned, and my bowel function is improving. And I've started walking too."

"Walking?" He looked up at me.

"Just a bit. In the parallel bars. I can walk nine meters now without stopping. But I still have to hold on with my left hand."

"That's remarkable." Dr. Chamberlain turned to Dr. Murray. "Do you remember the extent of her injury? Absolutely remarkable. We should do a case study on you. Motivation and recovery."

What? They hadn't expected me to recover? Even though they'd told me that my injury was incomplete? That motivation helped? I was glad I hadn't known.

"Let's see what we've got." Dr. Chamberlain clipped my X-rays to a backlit screen. "Everything looks good. We can get you out of that halo."

I glanced at Daniel. He smiled but looked anxious. I

wasn't, or at least I didn't think I was, but my legs and right arm were tremoring. Again, my body knew my feelings better than I did.

Dr. Chamberlain stood on one side of me, Dr. Murray on the other. They each inserted the head of a screwdriver in the bolts on either side of my forehead.

"Up for a race, Ken?" Dr. Chamberlain grinned.

Dr. Murray shook his head. "I don't think—"

"Ready, set, go!" Dr. Chamberlain shouted and the competition began. It was one that Dr. Chamberlain was sure to win. He had a power screwdriver; Dr. Murray did not.

Amazingly, it didn't hurt. Though it hadn't hurt when the nurses tightened the bolts on the halo every week either. It was as if my skull and flesh had remolded to accommodate the screws.

I only became aware of the blood as it trickled into my left eye.

"Stop! Richard! Stop!" Dr. Murray yelled over the drone of the power screwdriver. "She's bleeding. Stop!"

Dr. Chamberlain laid down his tool. "What happened?"

"Her hair got caught under the bolt. The more you twisted, the deeper it cut."

Dr. Chamberlain sat down at the desk, his face reddening as he jotted notes in my file. Dr. Murray gently removed the remaining screws from the back of my head. Together, they lifted the halo, freeing my neck and head. Dr. Murray swabbed the still bleeding hole on my forehead and covered it with a bandage. He fastened a collar around my neck. "You'll have to wear this for a week or so, until your neck muscles strengthen," he said. "The nurses will take off your vest when you get back to the rehab center."

"We'll see you again in about a month," Dr. Chamberlain said. "Keep up the good work."

Daniel was pale and silent as we headed back. The wheels creaked as the porter pushed the trolley.

"I should have said something!" Daniel said.

"What?"

"Back there. To that doctor. A race?"

"Don't worry about it."

"I can't believe I didn't say anything."

"It doesn't matter."

We continued down the hall, Daniel frowning, shaking his head.

"You need to lodge a formal complaint with the hospital administrator," he said when we returned to my room.

"I'm not doing that."

"Why not?"

"I don't want to."

"I will then."

"This is about me. Not you."

"I don't want him to get away with it."

"They saved my *life*. All I care about is that the halo is off and I'm getting better. That's it."

"I think you need to stand up for yourself."

"I don't want to argue about it."

"I don't know how you can tolerate this. I don't think I could."

"It would be harder for you. But I know what I'm doing. To get the best treatment, you have to know when to speak up and when to let things go. That's just how it is."

194

When he left, I rang for a nurse to remove the halo vest and transfer me to bed. I was tired. I needed to rest before lunch. What an ordeal! Had it been better or worse to have Daniel with me? Sometimes his presence smothered me. It was good to be alone again.

Until now, I'd thought Daniel and my father were nothing alike. But there was this: the struggle for space for myself when they were with me, the sense of relief when they were gone.

Once the nurse had settled me in bed, I rolled on my side. My head was right on the pillow, a cool softness against my cheek. Another patient had told me that when his halo had first been removed, his head felt like a meatball attached to his shoulders by a wet noodle, but so far, I just felt lighter and free. How long would it take for the holes in my forehead to fill in? Would I be scarred?

I closed my eyes and began tumbling toward sleep. I jolted awake. How would I sleep without suffocating myself? My head now nestled right into the pillow, no longer suspended in mid-air, a few inches above. Had I learned to sleep with my head on a pillow as a young child? Would my body remember how? Relax. Just relax. I had to trust that even in sleep, I'd look after myself.

NOVEMBER 25

FAT, WET SNOWFLAKES spiraled from the night sky, sparkling in the lamplight outside my window. The snow blanketed barren trees and carpeted the ground. Packing snow. I felt a thrill, like when I was a child and would whoop "snow" at the first flakes, anticipating snowmen, snow forts and angels, and skating and hot chocolate at the ice rink in front of the bandshell at Victoria Park.

Since my injury, everything seemed new: the yellow gold of sunflowers, the fresh snap of autumn air, the shifting shapes of clouds against a brilliant blue sky, and now this. Snow.

The snow accumulated. Ottawa winters were harsh: sub-zero temperatures, air so frigid each breath stung, uneven, icy sidewalks, and towering snowbanks at the curbside. How would I ever get a wheelchair through that?

And what about winter clothes? I could dress myself with one arm in T-shirts and pull-on shorts, running shoes with elasticized laces, but a down parka? Boots and gloves?

I wheeled to the intercom to ring for a nurse.

"Yes?"

"Can I get a transfer to bed?"

"Do you need two of us?"

"Only one. I can do a standing transfer now. I just need to be spotted."

"Be right there."

Mary, one of the weekend nurses, entered my room. She was plump with curly dark hair and freckled, pale skin. She was often a little disheveled, her nursing smock wrinkled or soiled. I liked her a lot.

"My goodness, look at you! When did the halo come off?"

"Almost two weeks ago. I guess I haven't seen you since then."

"Let's see this standing transfer. You keep getting better and better."

Mary stood nearby. I angled my chair by the side of the bed and applied the brakes. I leaned forward, braced my left hand on the arm of the chair, and pushed my weight through my legs to stand. I shuffled foot to foot to rotate then sat on the edge of the bed.

"Do you need a hand to lie down?"

"I can do that too!" I rolled a little on my hip and laid the right side of my upper body on the bed. I lifted my left leg from the floor and then my right so that my whole body was on the bed.

"That's terrific." She tucked the covers around me. "Not an easy thing to do."

"I hope I can transfer on my own soon. Without supervision."

"You're definitely heading in that direction."

"Would you mind putting some pain cream on my neck? There's a tube in my drawer. My neck really hurts since the halo came off. I try to ignore it, but…." It persisted: a burning ache in my neck muscles and snarls of pain that shot from the base of my skull to the top of my shoulders. The cream helped, a little.

"No problem." Mary reached into the drawer of the nightstand. "It takes a while for your neck to adjust. But it must feel good to be out of your halo. I know when my husband got his off, his mood really improved."

"Your husband was in a halo?"

"He's a quad. C4, complete. Has some movement in his hands. But not up and about like you." She winked. "We met here. Together almost three years now."

"Really?"

"We're looking to have a baby. Dr. Davis is helping us. Through the outpatient fertility program here. We've been talking about it for a while. At first, Harold, my husband, wasn't sure. Was worried about what kind of father he'd be. What he could give a child. Love, I told him. That's what he could give. And that baby would know him and love him too, just as he is."

But I understood Harold's concerns. The discrepancy between the life he'd anticipated before his injury and what he had now.

"Sweet dreams." She turned off the lights and closed the door.

Mary had fallen in love with a patient!

Love. And sex. I hadn't even thought about those things. My body was so fragile; I didn't want anyone near it. And right now, beyond improving physically and learning to do things on my own, I was almost completely devoid of desire. For anything at all.

My appetite was better, and I enjoyed some foods more than others, but I didn't much care what I ate. Nor did I care how I looked or what I wore. I ate for energy. I wore things that were easy for me to put on with one hand. My hair was in a ponytail so it wouldn't get in my way. Glasses had replaced contacts. And I could now put them on myself with one hand. Every day I tried to do something new on my own, but there was still a lot I couldn't do.

All I wanted was to be independent. I wanted to live on my own when I left here. I wanted to go back to school in the fall. All my energy was directed toward these goals. What had once seemed like a simple, basic existence consumed me now. Anything else was extraneous. I was firmly rooted in the present. And in my present, there were no frills. My life was reduced to rudimentary functions and working to regain them.

Would I love or be loved again? I couldn't even think about it. Right now, love and sex were vague concepts that would have to wait.

But I had wondered about children. A few weeks ago, I'd asked Martha whether I'd still be able to have children, if I wanted to. "Well," she'd said, "as you know, most women don't get their periods for months after their injuries, due to the shock. Though yours came back much earlier, of course. But once their periods return, women's fertility isn't affected by their spinal cord injuries. So, you'll be as fertile now as you were before the accident."

I had no idea how fertile I was. I'd never been pregnant, but I'd never had unprotected sex either. My mother's unusually direct and strident warnings, starting when I was about fourteen, had had their intended effect. "Whatever you do, do *not* get pregnant. Always use birth control. And if you do get pregnant, you *have* to have an abortion. You don't want to ruin your life." She'd said the same thing to my sister, but they were closer, so their discussion of this issue was less of a surprise. For my mom and I, it was an unusual bridge of the distance that had increased between us since my dad had left. And not until I was a few years older did I fully understand the reason behind my mother's concern.

Unlike women, men's fertility was affected by spinal cord injuries. They might have erectile dysfunction and low sperm counts. Martha had told me that too. That was why they'd established the fertility program at the rehab center. Luckily for Harold and Mary.

I shut my eyes, falling asleep to the image of a man in his thirties, seated in a power chair, cradling an infant on his lap.

■ ■ ■

On Monday when Martha brought in my breakfast tray, I asked, "Do you know Mary? She works weekends?"

"Sure."

"So, you know she married a patient?"

"A few of the nurses have. Even our supervisor did. But mostly that doesn't happen now."

"Why not?"

"It's not really ethical and...well...there was an incident. Not here. At another hospital. Maybe in Toronto. I'm not sure."

"What happened?"

Martha blushed. "I really shouldn't say."

"Come on. Tell me."

"It was terrible really." She stifled a giggle. "It's a sin to laugh."

"What happened?"

"One of the patients broke his pelvis. During the...act."

"What?"

"He was having a relationship with one of the nurses. At some point, during the night shift, well, I guess she got right on top of him. And then it happened. She got fired. Thankfully, he healed up okay in the end."

"That's wild." So funny, tragic, and human, all at the same time.

"Since then, there've been tighter controls. No relationships with inpatients, for sure. And it's discouraged on the outside too."

Of course, that was the right thing to do, but Mary glowed when she spoke of Harold and of getting pregnant. There was so little joy here. Shouldn't any possibility of happiness be allowed?

NOVEMBER 28

AT ONE END of the parallel bars, I parked my wheelchair and locked the brakes. As I was about to stand, Sheila held up a four-legged cane with a broad base.

"Let's try this today," she said. "It's a quad cane. You can start by using it as you walk between the bars, so you'll feel safe."

"You think I'm ready?"

"You can let go of the cane and grab the bar if you get nervous. And I'll be right behind you with your chair. First, I'll show you how to use it." She switched the cane from her right to left hand, lifted it, moved it forward about the length of a step, and placed it on the ground ahead of her left foot. "Now I step with my right, then the left. Then cane, then right, then left. Got it?"

"I've got it." I hadn't realized that walking with a cane was something to be learned. I'd never even thought about it, but then again, I hadn't had to, until now. And now I felt excited that I was ready to learn.

I stood and grasped the handle of the cane with my left hand. I leaned on it a little, and it held my weight. Stable. My stomach fluttered as I swung it forward, then stepped with my right foot and then my left. "There!" My first independent steps! Then again. Cane. Right. Left. Cane. Right. Left. I stopped after a few steps. "This is fantastic. I'm really walking now!"

"See if you can make it to the end," Sheila said behind me.

I felt steady, comfortable as I walked. Cane. Right. Left. Cane. Right. Left. When I reached the end of the bars, I sank back into my wheelchair. My right leg trembled slightly with a spasm, but it stopped when I pushed my foot against the floor.

"How do you feel?" Sheila asked.

"Excellent. Not that tired."

"Take a rest. Then we can try a few steps outside the bars."

After I drank some water, we moved to the center of the room. It was a quiet afternoon. Only one other physiotherapist stretched a patient on a plinth in the far corner. Good. I needed to concentrate fully with no distractions. Taking a few steps with the cane eclipsed any goal, any other achievement I'd had in my previous life. I ached to succeed.

I parked my chair, pushed off the armrest with my left hand, and stood, taking the cane in my hand. Cane. Right. Left. That was all I had to do.

"I'll follow you with your chair," Sheila said. "Ready?"

I edged the cane forward. Scanned the room, my place in it. Space. Unending, open space swirled around me. Nothing but the cane and my own body to hold me up, to withstand gravity, to balance myself on a spinning planet, an ant on a gumball, teetering. Blood beat in my ears. The floor tilted, rushed toward me. The walls, the ceiling, closed in. My right leg shuddered. I was frozen. Couldn't move.

"It's okay, Susan. Just shift onto your right foot to stop the spasm, then go. I'm right here," Sheila's voice broke through.

I weighted my right foot. The shaking ceased. Go. Just go. Don't surrender. I riveted my eyes to my feet. Don't look anywhere else. Go!

"Cane. Right," I whispered as I extended my right leg forward. A small, shaky, first step. "Left." I stepped with the left. Now. Again. "Cane. Right. Left," I said, this time with more force. "Cane. Right. Left."

Sheila's voice joined mine and together we chanted: "Cane. Right. Left. Cane. Right. Left." Ten steps! I collapsed in my wheelchair, almost sick with relief. I hadn't been defeated. With Sheila's help, I'd triumphed!

NOVEMBER 29

AFTER MARTHA HAD cleared away my lunch tray, I sat in my wheelchair waiting. Waiting for Gary to arrive for a visit before I went to OT. Waiting and going to appointments. That was my life now. Waiting and waiting. I just wanted to get better, for this part of my life to be over, so I could begin again. But for now, there was this. The endless waiting. And Gary was late.

At almost 1:30, Gary bounced into the room. "Afternoon, sweetie," he said. I hadn't seen him in a few weeks. He still called to check in every couple of days, but things had cooled between us since my visit to his apartment. On the phone yesterday, he'd mentioned that he'd just returned from a wellness retreat recommended by his counselor Joanne.

I was skeptical of anything endorsed by Joanne. A couple of my friends at work had been assigned to her when they'd requested therapy through the employee-assistance program. One had described an office replete with dream catchers, crystals, and shelves of self-help books from the 1970s. Another had said that Joanne had done a rune stone casting with her as part of a goal-setting exercise.

I hadn't fared much better when I'd sought counseling through the program after I separated from Daniel. Near the end of my second appointment, Sylvie, a young, petite French-Canadian woman who seemed to be a less experienced therapist than I was, informed me that we didn't need to meet anymore. I'd been through a lot already in my life and was obviously a strong person with good coping skills. I just needed to get out more. "Go see a foreign film at the ByTowne," she'd said, "and after go to the burger place across the street and have a 'fry.' You'll be fine." But I wasn't. I wasn't fine at all.

Gary dragged a chair across the room and sat beside me at the window. "You're looking great. What have you been up to?"

"Yesterday I started walking with a cane. Just a few steps. And I need to be spotted, but still…."

"That's wonderful. Onward and upward." He winked. "Soon you'll be good as new."

"Not *quite.*"

"Want to go for a stroll in the hallway later?"

"I don't have much time. I have OT at two o'clock."

"Sorry. I guess I was a little late."

"That's okay. How was your retreat?"

His eyes shone. "Completely changed my life."

"Really?"

"You should do it too. I mean, when you're better."

"What was it like?"

"There were about fifty of us. We all stayed for five nights at a hotel near the airport. During the day we had workshops on different topics, all aimed at self-understanding and growth, things like being self 'full,' not self 'less.' The speakers were really dynamic. And every night we wrote all our thoughts, feelings, and experiences in a journal. It was intense. Sometimes, I was up most of the night. Then we processed them together in small groups the next morning.

"The most important thing I learned," Gary said, "is to remain in the present zone. Stay in the here and now. The last night was the best. We had a big celebration called the Pageant of Rebirth. Everyone got up on stage and sang a song that they'd picked with the help of their group leader to represent their new self. Guess what my song was?"

"I have no idea."

"Soul Man." Gary sang a few bars. "Everyone cheered. It was magical."

"It sounds like a cult. How much did you pay for this?"

"Three thousand bucks, but my extended health care insurance covered the cost. As medical treatment while I'm on stress leave. And it's not like a cult at all. It's about creating a community. These are the nicest, warmest people I've ever met. Everyone understood what I've been through, and they encouraged me to stay strong."

"Oh?"

"I can't describe how good it feels to be part of something like this. We'll even continue to meet regularly for fellowship. I'm hosting my first group soon." He smiled shyly. "I have something important to tell you. I hope you'll be happy for me."

"What?"

"I met someone at the retreat."

"What do you mean?"

"We've only been out a few times, but I can feel it's something special. A bond that's growing deep."

"What?" My stomach was a tight fist. I felt like I might throw up.

"She understands I still need to come here. She supports my sense of responsibility."

"What? How could you...already?"

"You said you just want to be friends. And you're moving back to Toronto."

"That's not the point." My legs trembled. "You've never even apologized for the accident. Not once have you said you were sorry for what happened to me. And now, this?"

Gary stared at the floor. "There was nothing I could have done. The moose came out of nowhere." He glanced up. "Of course, I'm sorry about your injury. But it wasn't my fault. And one thing I learned at the retreat was I have to move on. Take care of myself.... I'm sorry, but I do."

"I want you out of here. *Now.*"

"I think we need to talk about this. I didn't realize you'd be so upset."

"Get out. Just get out of here!"

He headed to the door. "I'll call you tomorrow. Once you've had a chance to process this, you'll see it's for the best."

Every cell of my body exploded with rage. How could he start dating someone else? How dare he "move on" while I was stuck here?

DECEMBER 8

I CHECKED THE CLOCK. Five to seven. Almost time. My mom wasn't due back until eight o'clock and then we'd have peppermint tea before I had to start getting ready for bed. I glanced at the phone. Almost time.

I had to stop. I knew I did, but every night for almost a week at seven-fifteen, there was this. As the minutes clicked by, I'd get jumpy anticipating the call, fidgeting, impatient for my "fix."

I hadn't really planned it. It had just happened after Gary's last visit, following his attempts to contact me.

The first time he'd called, the day after sharing the news about his girlfriend, I'd hung up at the sound of his voice. When he called the next day, I'd reached a decision. Pausing after he said hello, I told him I never wanted to hear from him again. "Don't call. Don't come here. I want you out of my life."

I thought he might persist. He didn't.

But I couldn't let go. I kept picturing Gary and this woman skiing, hiking in the Gatineau, strolling through the market, having cozy dinners in restaurants, stopping in cafés.

A world now denied to me, but not *him*.

"You seem distracted," my mother had said.

"I'm just tired. Maybe I'm getting a cold."

So easy for Gary to step out of the car and into a new life. In that same car my body had been destroyed. I would carry this reminder of our relationship forever. He was free to forget.

Then a couple of nights after our final phone call, rage burgeoned within me. I envisioned a candlelit supper, the happy couple snuggled on the couch watching TV. How dare he discard me?

I punched in star sixty-seven to block call display and then Gary's number. The line engaged. Two, three, four times it rang. "Hel-lo-o," a chipper Gary answered. I slammed down the receiver, waited fifteen minutes, and redialed. By the third call, he sounded irritated. "Who is this?"

I wheeled away from the phone. At least I could disrupt what I couldn't destroy.

Calm settled over me. A quiet calm. A familiar relief. Reminding me how I'd felt as a teenager after I'd cut myself. For four, maybe five years, I'd done it. At least once a week, sometimes more. A dark fury would mount, seeking release.

I remembered a dusky evening in mid-December, a few months before my sixteenth birthday after a "visit" with Mr. Semple in an isolated parking lot at Gibbons Park. Blotting himself with a tissue, zipping his fly, he turned the keys in the ignition. "Better get home to the family. Almost suppertime. Where can I drop you?"

"The library."

When he pulled over on Queens Avenue, I'd jumped out

of the car and raced up the steps to the double doors of the main entrance. Comforted by the hot dry air, the musty scent of books, of pages, of words. My refuge. My better home. I rushed to the basement, past the children's section and the AV room. Safe. I just wanted to be safe. At the vending machine, I inserted a quarter to dispense a lukewarm, watery coffee in a thin plastic cup. Each sip dispelled the salty, egg-white residue in my mouth. I extracted a pubic hair that had snagged between my teeth. Gray. *Yuck.*

I no longer felt like an adventurous heroine in a novel, but kind of icky, kind of used. And yet there was still something...something about being chosen...about being wanted that I couldn't quite give up.

A tension rose from deep inside, like a prelude to an outburst of screams or sobs, but I was silent, my eyes dry.

The women's washroom was vacant. I slammed the door and bolted my favorite stall, the one on the end, by the green, puke-colored wall. I put down my knapsack and settled on the toilet seat. Safe. Alone and safe.

The outer door creaked open. Someone else had entered. I grabbed my bag from the floor, tucked my knees to my chest and breathed softly. Quiet, as if no one were here. Then the flush, the running tap, the click of the hand dryer. The banging door. Good. Alone again.

I scrunched up the sleeves of my sweater and examined my forearms. Smooth flesh, like a blank page. Upon closer inspection, a few thin white scars.

I fished a package of razor blades out of my backpack. The steel edge was cold against my skin. I made my first line straight, about an inch long. The pressure gentle but firm.

Deep enough to leave a scar, but superficial enough so the blood would clot quickly. Blood seeped from the opening: a thin red line. The knot within me eased. I drew another line with the razor's edge. The blood pooled. A perfect *X*. One by one, I carved two more *X*s in my left arm, in the skin above the wrist, below the elbow. The oozing blood was a tonic. My mind started to clear. I felt light and pure.

Just like I did now, fifteen years later in my hospital room.

The next night I repeated the calls, the hang-ups. And once again, my actions alleviated my torment like a balm.

I refocused my efforts on rehab. "You seem much better," my mother said. And I was. I limited myself to three calls a night, at ten-minute intervals. Sometimes I'd get the answering machine, other times Gary, and a few times Crystal, who'd once screamed, "Stop calling here! Leave us alone!"

They likely suspected me but couldn't prove anything.

The clock's hands reached seven-fifteen. It was time.

Two, three, four rings. "Hello?" Gary bellowed over the clamor of voices in the background. I hung up quickly. Was he having a party? With his new girlfriend? His new cult friends? I watched the clock, restraining myself to observe the full ten minutes before my next call.

"Susan?" Gary identified me for the first time. Panicked, I replaced the receiver. Less than a minute later, my telephone rang. I had to answer, otherwise the call would be redirected to the nursing station, and they would come into my room, curious.

"Please don't hang up," Gary said.

I remained silent, waiting.

"I'm hosting a fellowship meeting tonight. We all

understand your pain, but this has to stop. We're all here for you. Can you tell us how to help?"

My cheeks flamed. A room full of people, their pity and disgust, discussing the poor, crippled girl. How to cope with her, what to do. "I'll stop," I said and quickly hung up.

What was wrong with me? This shameful compulsion. Was I falling apart?

I didn't even want to be with Gary. I really didn't. But he'd found someone else so easily. What if I never did?

I had to regain control. An image from my high school physics class came to me. Iron filings scattered on a piece of paper, the tiny fragments clustered at the end of a magnet waved over them, becoming a solid clump, held together by the invisible force. I too could take what had been shattered and become strong and whole.

DECEMBER 10

"I THOUGHT WE MIGHT take a little drive today," my mom said. "If you're up to it? It might be a nice change."

"Okay," I said. Shortly after the doctors removed my halo, Barb, my occupational therapist, had taught me how to transfer from my wheelchair to the passenger seat of my mother's car. I was no longer restricted to using the accessible bus, but I hadn't left the rehab center since then. I hadn't really wanted to.

My mother parked in front of the rehab center where the pavement was clear of ice and snow. She jumped out and opened the passenger door. I wheeled down the ramp, angled my chair between the open door and the seat, and applied the brakes to my chair.

My mom moved into help. "I want to see if I can do it myself."

"I'll be right here if you need me."

I pushed myself up to stand, grasped the car door for balance, took a few small steps to pivot, then plopped down into the seat, sideways, my legs still outside the car. "Almost there."

"You're doing great."

I rotated my upper body, placed my left foot on the floor in front of me, then used my left hand to lift and guide my right leg beside it. "There." I exhaled, unaware I'd been holding my breath. "I did it."

"You want a hand with the seatbelt?"

"Yes. I'll have to work up to that." So much effort. It was hard to believe that a few months ago I could just hop into a car.

"Where do you want to go?" My mother turned the keys in the ignition.

"Um…," but as the car started, with the vibration of the engine, my stomach clenched, and the taste of a rusted penny flooded my mouth. The car was so much smaller than the accessible bus. I felt more vulnerable, more exposed. As the vehicle shifted forward, my right leg jumped and my right arm shook with a spasm.

"Maybe by the Parliament Buildings, then down the canal to Dow's Lake?" My voice cracked, but I couldn't give in to the fear. I had to be able to do this.

My mom drove along, chatting about our upcoming plans for Christmas and Kathryn's visit. But I wasn't listening. My eyes were riveted to the road, on other cars and drivers. Each time my mother stopped at a red light, or made a left turn, I saw only the potential skid, the crunch of the collision, the crush from behind. I couldn't stop myself. If I'd been paying more attention in Gary's car that night, maybe none of this would have happened.

If I'd known there were moose along that stretch of highway, I'd never have suggested going at night, or at least I would have been vigilant, scanning the forested embankments, the sides of the road for their glowing red eyes lit up by the flare of the headlights.

If only…. If only….

I tried not to think about it. What could have happened. What I could have changed. Too painful and pointless, a random occurrence, the outcome couldn't be altered. I was here, now, like this. And yet…there remained a small space where I'd had a shred of control, a slim possibility that my attentiveness could have had an impact, so I was alert to other cars, other drivers. From now on, as far as possible, I'd control what I could.

"Did you hear me?" My mom pulled into a parking spot in front of a café.

"Sorry. What?"

"Did you want to go in for a coffee?"

"You mean leave the car? Go in with my wheelchair? No."

"Are you sure? It might be fun."

"I don't want to. Not yet."

"We'll go whenever you're ready."

I stared at my lap. Before the accident when I saw people using wheelchairs in public, I'd thought nothing of it. Why did I think it was different for me? But I didn't want to go in. I just wanted to go back to the rehab center. To be safe and hidden in my room, unexposed.

DECEMBER 15

"HOW'S IT GOING?" Sheila asked, joining me at the standing frame. The frame resembled a podium. My arms rested on a tray, knee-level cuffs held my legs in place, and my feet were strapped to the base. The frame supported me so I could stand, bearing my full weight, for a longer period of time than I could walk. Sheila had said it would help strengthen my legs.

"Fine," I said. "Just a few more minutes before I work out with Kyle."

"What do you have there?"

I dropped the pen clutched in my left hand, picked up my workbook from the tray, and passed it to her. "I'm teaching myself to write with my left hand. I was right-handed before so…."

Sheila flipped to the bright red cover. A grinning child clasped a bouquet of balloons and the title *Writing Is Fun!* was emblazoned in yellow script across the top.

"I got my mom to buy it," I said. "I figured if it worked the first time…."

"That's a great idea." She studied the page where I'd traced, then copied the letters between faintly printed lines: *AAAAAAAA…aaaaaaaa…BBBBBBBB.*

"It looks good." She returned the book to the tray. "One day you're writing your dissertation…." She shook her head. "And the next day—"

"Unbelievable, isn't it?" I forced a half-smile but blinked back sudden tears.

I knew Sheila hadn't intended to hurt me, but her comment cut through all my defenses. Compared to being completely paralyzed, every action, every movement, and every improvement was a triumph. I concentrated on the next achievement. Sometimes I forgot how much I had lost and how far I still had to go.

The timer buzzed. My twenty minutes of standing were over.

"Be right there," Kyle called from the other side of the room. When he reached me, he grabbed my wheelchair and positioned it behind me. "Want to start with arms or legs?" he asked, as I sat back into the chair.

"Arms, I guess." Though really, I could only do one arm, my left one. My right arm was no longer flaccid, but involuntary spasticity caused the fingers to curl into a fist and the elbow to remain bent at ninety degrees most of the time.

I parked in a corner near the free weight area.

"Two pounds for biceps curls?" Kyle asked.

"That's what we did last time."

"You want to try three today?"

"Yes." I took the weight from Kyle and began the reps.

A few minutes later, a good-looking guy in his late teens wheeled into the room.

"Afternoon, Michel," Kyle said.

"Hey, Kyle," Michel said and nodded in my direction.

"Hi." I'd seen him around but didn't know him. He wasn't part of the spinal cord program.

Kyle set Michel up at a pulley system. Michel held the grip firmly with his left hand and tugged the cable. "I can handle more weight than this."

"Sure thing, buddy." Kyle adjusted the weights. "Try that."

Michel had black curly hair and soft brown eyes. His build was athletic, and I imagined he'd played a lot of sports...*before.* But now his right lower leg was encased in a metal frame with pins and screws extending into his shin. It reminded me of my halo.

Michel grunted as he pulled the cable across his chest. His torso torqued with the effort, causing the T-shirt sleeve on his right shoulder to flap loosely in the air, empty where his arm should have been.

"Ready for the foot cycle, Susan?" Kyle asked.

"Sure."

After removing the footrest, Kyle attached the apparatus to the bottom of my wheelchair and strapped my feet onto the pedals. I loved the foot cycle. It gave me the sensation of riding a bike and I was able to move my legs faster doing this than anything else.

"Can I try fifteen minutes today?" I asked.

"No problem." He set the timer. "Just let me know if you get tired."

My attention drifted back to Michel. His damage was only on the right. Some type of accident. Car or motorcycle most likely. Maybe he'd been the passenger, side-swiped by another vehicle, crumpled metal pulverizing his shin, shearing off his arm.

I continued to pedal. If it were possible, would I trade places with Michel? He'd probably walk almost normally after his leg healed and would eventually be using a prosthetic arm. No neurological complications, no useless appendages, but an absence. What would that be like?

"Can I get some water?" Michel released the pulley. "*Whew.* That was hard work, man."

"Here you go." Kyle handed him a cone-shaped paper cup.

He gulped it down. "Another?"

Kyle returned with a plastic mug full of water.

"Check out my watch." Michel thrust out his arm.

"That's pretty cool," Kyle said.

"I got it yesterday. My brother and I went to the St. Laurent Centre."

He'd gone to the mall? Like that?

"It was great to get out of here," Michel continued. "We had an awesome time. All the crowds, everything decorated for Christmas, the kids lined up to see Santa. Burgers and shakes in the food court. I can't wait to go back."

Wow! Even with my halo off, I didn't want to be displayed in public, had refused to go into a quiet café with my mother last weekend. But Michel hadn't just gone out; he'd celebrated.

I glanced at Michel. Kyle was adjusting the pulley for him. They both started chuckling over a shared joke. Why couldn't I be more like Michel? Less self-conscious, able to go out in the world no matter how I looked. He didn't care.

Why did I?

I flashed to a telephone conversation I'd had with my grandmother a few days ago.

"I'm walking now with a cane…."

"Walking?" She had gasped.

"Yes! Can you believe it? It's fantastic that I can do it. All on my own. Just short distances, but—"

"My word! It's incredible. When I think what you've been through…." Her voice trembled.

"It's okay, Grandma. I really am getting better."

"It's a miracle. A blessing from God. You know a lot of people are praying for you?"

"I know. It's very kind."

"You remember Betty, from across the hall? Her whole church prayed for you. Many times. And they're *Baptists*."

"Oh?" I was unsure how to interpret the emphasis.

"Imagine what they would think if some day you walked right in there. Right up the aisle to the front of the congregation. For all to see."

"I'm not doing that." I suppressed a giggle.

"For land sakes, why not?"

"I'd feel very uncomfortable."

"Think what it would mean to them. They'd think so much of you."

"I *am* grateful that they prayed for me. But I'm not doing that."

"Oh…." She clicked her tongue. "Maybe you'll change your mind."

In my head, I often heard my grandma, my mother, Daniel, and sometimes even my father: Don't wear that dress.

Don't put your hair behind your ears. Don't slouch. Don't do that. Don't say that. Don't look like that. Don't be like that. All my life, two extremes: I was either invisible or being scrutinized and never quite measuring up.

Michel was now doing triceps extensions with a dumbbell. I imagined him laughing and talking as his brother wheeled him in and out of stores and helped him try on watches. He just wanted to have fun and be happy. He didn't seem to be worried about what other people thought. I needed to change. I needed to be more like him.

DECEMBER 20

"MOM. STOP PACING." She'd crossed the room, back and forth, about ten times. Her anxiety was contagious.

"I'm not." She paused in mid-stride. "Why would you say that?"

"Just sit down. Are you nervous?"

"I'm thinking of everything I have to do." She drummed her fingers on the armrest of the chair. "Are you sure an hour is enough time to get to the airport? With having to park and everything?"

"More than enough time. It's not a big airport. Or very busy."

"But it's the holidays."

"If you're worried, leave now."

"I'm sure you know how long it takes. I'll wait a few minutes."

"Are you going to come right back here once you pick up Kathryn?"

"Yes. Are you all packed?"

"Over there." I pointed to a knapsack in the corner. "Martha and I did it this morning."

"Are you sure you have everything? Do you want me to check?"

"I have everything. Besides, I'm just going home." Home. Incredibly, I was going home.

"I can always run over here if you need something. I still have a lot of errands to do. I have to pick up the turkey and do a bit more shopping. You *still* haven't told me what you want for Christmas."

"I want to be able to walk. I don't care about anything else."

"You have to have presents to open under the tree. I've gotten a few things but—"

"Get me a sweater."

"What color?"

"I don't know, Mom. Black. I'm happy just to be coming home. And that Kathryn is going to be here."

"I want everything to be nice."

"I know."

"I'd better go. See you in a couple of hours."

Christmas. I'd hated it for years. Though there *had* been some good times, way back. When Kathryn was a little girl and would crawl into my bed at four in the morning, her excitement barely contained, as we'd creep into the living room to open our stockings, whispering together, trying not to wake up anyone else.

But mostly my memories of it melded together, leaving impressions of misery and dread. The house stuffy and overheated to prevent our grandparents from getting cold, an explosion of gifts under the tree, overfilled stockings.

Kathryn and I would tear off the wrappings from an

endless succession of presents, and our grandfather would reminisce about Christmas morning when he was a boy, the thrill of an orange and a few walnuts in a sock. Our grandmother's tight-lipped smile would fail to hide her disapproval, the certainty that come January, they would be footing the bill for my mother's extravagance.

By the time I was a teenager, I'd started insisting that my mother return some of my gifts. I felt suffocated by the volume of presents that she couldn't afford, but there was something more. A refusal to be complicit, to pretend that this display somehow nullified the reality of the other three hundred and sixty-four days of the year, or at least made them easier to forget.

After the presents, the day would yawn on. My mom sipped vodka from a coffee mug, and my grandpa snuck out to the garage for swigs of brandy and clandestine cigarettes. My mother and grandmother bickered in the kitchen over how much sage to put in the stuffing, how much milk to add to the mashed potatoes, and how long to cook the "bird."

By five o'clock we'd be seated at the table. After grace, plates would be passed, the conversation a never-ending tirade about the inadequacy of the meal.

"I've simply ruined it," my grandmother would say. "This gravy has lumps of flour and no flavor. Absolutely no flavor."

"It's perfect, Mom," my mother would say. "You make the best gravy. The turkey is the problem. I overcooked it. It's too dry."

Everything was delicious, but the food stuck in my throat. The moment the last mouthful of pumpkin pie was swallowed, I'd leap from the table, clear the dishes, and retreat to my room, relieved to shut myself in and everyone else out. I'd lie on the bed, immersed in a book, peeling brightly colored foil off chocolate balls, popping one after another into my mouth.

This year, though, I was looking forward to the holidays. Over two weeks away from the rehab center, and I'd actually be in my own home. Over the past month, the insurance company had arranged to adapt my apartment so that it would be accessible. Last week, the rehab consultant had confirmed it was ready and I could go home for Christmas. A wheelchair lift had been installed for the steps at the entrance. There were bars in the bathroom, a bath bench, and a raised toilet seat. Finally, I had somewhere else I could be, a place of my own. I couldn't wait!

If only my mother could relax more, quiet her intensity about the gifts, the tree, the food, stop trying to make everything perfect, and believe me when I insisted that it didn't matter. This push and pull between us—my mother's relentless efforts—overwhelmed me and made me want to withdraw. The tendrils of the past encroached into the present. Maybe it was an unavoidable part of our relationship. Maybe my mother couldn't let go, and maybe neither could I.

■ ■ ■

In the few minutes it took me to wheel from the entrance of the rehab center to my mother's car parked out front, the cold had penetrated me: biting the exposed skin on my cheeks and stinging my nostrils with each breath. Kathryn opened the passenger door and I put the brakes on the chair, then stood, transferring myself to the front seat. It was even easier than when I'd done it almost two weeks ago.

"You are *so* much better." Kathryn hugged me as she leaned over to fasten my seatbelt. "I can't believe it."

"I just hope it continues. I'm so happy you're here."

"Me too." Kathryn squeezed my shoulder as she climbed into the back.

My mom slammed the trunk shut and slid into the driver's seat. "We've got your chair, your cane, your clothes, and meds. I think we're all set." She started the car and pulled away from the building.

"Your cane?" Kathryn said. "I didn't know you were using it that much."

"I'm using it more and more. I'm hoping I can practice with it a lot over the holidays. See how independent I can be at home." At home. I was really going to be in my own apartment. Having Christmas with my family. Like a regular person with a regular life. No appointments, no routines, no nurses barging in. I could do what I wanted, when I wanted.

Last week when Lisa was visiting me in the hospital, she and my mom were in my room. It was almost ten o'clock at night, we were drinking peppermint tea and watching a video of *Absolutely Fabulous* on the small TV my mom had brought in for me. Fun. We were actually having fun. Then the rap on the door and a nurse I didn't know entered. "Visiting hours are over. Time for your guests to leave. It's bedtime."

"But—" I said.

"I'll be back to turn out your lights in ten minutes," the nurse said, her clipped steps exiting my room.

Her intrusion, her reprimand, it was like she'd punched

me in the stomach. I opened my mouth, but only a ragged sob escaped. Tears poured from me, I gulped for air, suddenly overcome. "Why…why can't they just leave me alone?" Something in me unraveled, and I cried even harder.

"It's okay, honey," my mom said, patting my arm. "I know it's awful, but we'll finish watching the show tomorrow."

"We're not bothering anybody. The volume is low. It's just their rules," Lisa said.

"I know," I said, trying to swallow my sobs. I didn't want that nurse to know that she'd shattered me. I had to calm down by the time she returned. "It's just…like they are taking everything away."

It was my first real cry since the accident. But it hadn't been the "good" cry several nurses had claimed I needed. I felt defeated, as if something had been torn from me. Something I wanted back.

Every day I struggled to stay positive, to work as hard as I could on my recovery. Complete paralysis was my baseline, so I celebrated every physical improvement, every new thing I could do for myself. But to do this I needed to shield myself from loss, the loss of control over my body, the loss of control over my life. The nurse with her patronizing commands had broken through and I was devastated. Despite all the gains, I was forced to admit that in many ways I remained powerless, lacked the freedom to even decide when to turn off the TV, when to ask my mom and Lisa to leave, or when to go to bed.

My mother turned onto the main road, exiting the hospital grounds. I was so happy to be getting out of there, at least for a little while.

"Turn up the heat, Mom," Kathryn said. "It's freezing."

"Must be a change from Vancouver," I said. "I hope you brought a warm coat."

"It's nice to see the sun, though," Kathryn said.

And it was. From a cerulean sky, the sun glittered on the piled banks, snow packed hard against the pavement, the layers left behind by plows or shovels. It was the kind of snow that squeaked like Styrofoam under your boots as you walked. Would I ever hear that sound again?

As we drove along, I half-listened as my mom and Kathryn talked, occasionally murmuring a response. More at ease than last time in the car, I was still alert but allowed some of my attention to be drawn to the action on the streets.

We stopped at a red light before crossing the bridge over the canal, and I watched the skaters below: pink, red, yellow, green, and blue, toques and ski jackets, a fluid ribbon of color against white. Steam spewed from the small wooden huts dotting the banks selling hot chocolate and beaver tails, the sugary pastry made tart with squirts of lemon. Those were my favorite.

I'd bought new skates at an end of season sale last March. I hadn't used them and now probably never would. I turned away from the window.

"Susan?" my mother asked. "Is that okay with you?"

"What?"

"Swiss Chalet for dinner?"

"Sure."

"We can't get it in Vancouver," Kathryn said. "It's funny what you miss."

"Here we are." My mother swung into the driveway. "Home."

While Kathryn fetched the wheelchair from the trunk, I checked out the renovations. My apartment occupied the lower level of a red brick duplex. The entrance was at the side of the house where four stairs led to a covered verandah made of gray wood. A shiny metal lift had been cut into the steps, just large enough for me in my wheelchair.

"Do you want some help?" Kathryn asked after I'd transferred to my chair.

"I want to see if I can do it myself." Before the holidays, Dr. Davis had given me a discharge date: January 31. This vacation was a trial run. I needed to see what I could and couldn't manage on my own, what might still have to be altered, and what I might have to hire an attendant to do. My mom was going to stay with me for the first week of February, but after that, I'd be on my own.

The driveway was well cleared of snow and ice, and I moved easily into the lift. I depressed the button and with a mechanical whirring, slowly rose to the porch.

I wheeled to the door. "Mom, can you give me the keys? I want to try this too."

Removing my left mitten with my teeth, I reached up, unlocked the door, and turned the knob to open it wide. I kicked my left leg forward and propelled myself over a small lip in the doorway that I'd never noticed before. I was in!

While my mom and Kathryn unloaded the car, I struggled with my coat. I tugged the right sleeve with my left hand and pulled off the left sleeve with my mouth. I wriggled out and flung the jacket on a chair.

Home, my home, yet everything seemed unfamiliar. It smelled like my mother's house, a mixture of cleaning solutions and hair products. Not an unpleasant odor, but also not mine. The living–dining room area was stark: a futon couch, a TV on a black plywood stand, a desk, a computer, a small bookcase, a wooden table, and a few chairs. My posters—the Kandinsky and Van Gogh's *Irises*—hung in my hospital room, which was full of my things. But here, there was only absence. A default apartment, for a default life.

My mom lugged in a bag of groceries. "Feel good to be home, honey?"

"Yes. Of course." I knew that was what she wanted to hear. And it did feel good to be out of the rehab center, the way I imagined a captive might feel after being released. But I felt like a stranger. Like I'd stumbled into someone else's life, the apartment of a missing person or a murder victim, and I was a detective searching for clues, trying to deduce the kind of person who had lived here, what their life had been like.

Kathryn dragged in her suitcase. "That's the last of it."

"Great," my mother said. "I'm just going to run out and get the chicken. I won't be long."

After my sister had put everything away, she pulled out a chair and sat beside me at the table. "Can I get you anything?" She stifled a yawn.

"I'm good. You seem tired."

"I was up at four this morning. So I am, kind of."

"Why don't you lie down in my room? I'll wake you up when Mom gets back."

"Are you sure?"

"I'll be fine. We have lots of time to visit."

"Maybe I will." Kathryn stretched up to stand. She

unfastened the tiny ivory buttons of her beige cardigan and shrugged it off, then unlatched a thin silver chain at the back of her neck and set it on the table. Her actions were so deft, so quick, unfaltering. I could hardly believe it. Had I ever moved so freely? Had it ever been possible?

Once Kathryn left, I unlocked the brakes of my chair and wheeled to the kitchen. I opened the fridge, reached inside, grabbed a liter of milk, and put it back in. I tugged at the oven door and extended my left arm to see if I could reach the controls for the burners at the back of the stove. I slid the cutlery drawers open and shut.

I stood and opened a cupboard and studied the arrangement of plates and bowls, glasses and cups. I tested the weight of a dinner plate, thick white and heavy ceramic. I'd need to get some lighter dishes, at least for a while.

I returned to my chair and rolled into the bathroom. The doorway was wide enough for me to pass through.

I transferred on and off the toilet then wheeled to the bathtub: bath bench, hand-held shower, grab bars, a non-slip mat. It was almost identical to the bathtub I used at the rehab center.

So far everything seemed manageable. It looked like I really would be able to return here and live on my own.

Back in the kitchen, I turned on the tap and filled a glass with water. Another success. Maybe tomorrow I'd try to make a simple meal: a sandwich or fruit and yogurt. I headed into the living room and the water jiggled with the wheelchair's movements, a little spilled in my lap. Next time, I wouldn't fill the glass so full.

At my desk, I set down the water and opened the drawer.

On top of a pile of papers was a copy of my dissertation proposal, the draft I'd completed a few days before the accident. I set it aside. I'd look at it later when I was back for good. I dug deeper and found a few loose papers and a notebook. I peeked inside and found a to-do list and a budget I'd roughed out for the summer. I startled as if a jolt of electricity coursed through me. My right arm shook, but I couldn't look away. I clasped my right arm with my left hand to still it. I examined each letter, each number. *My* handwriting. I tried to connect to the person who'd written this. Tried to imagine *her* thoughts, *her* feelings, *her* movements from that time. It was impossible. The distance was eerie.

I'd never again be the person who'd penned these notes. I'd left on a Sunday afternoon in August, planning to spend two weeks hiking in the mountains and then return, tanned and more relaxed. I could never have imagined that that night my body, my life, would be fractured, and I wouldn't be back for four months.

Four months of near death, almost complete paralysis, total dependence. Four months of gradual recovery, a working left arm, staggered walking with a cane, a return of some function, of some independence. Four months later, I had become this. Whatever *this* turned out to be.

Multiple selves. Not the self who had last left this apartment, locked the door, eager for a holiday. Not the self who had lain motionless in a halo, tubes replacing bodily functions. Not even the self I was twenty minutes ago, before I had come home, to be confronted by this now-unfamiliar space, these startling remnants of my previous life.

Until now, I'd thought that recovery was a reclamation, a return to self. But it wasn't. And I would have to go forward now as I was, as best I could, and try to live again.

JANUARY 4, 1996

ON MY FIRST DAY back after the holidays, a repugnant familiarity flooded my senses when I entered the lobby of the rehab center. The stale air, not quite medicinal but institutional, was hot and oppressive. Outpatients gathered in the reception area, waiting for appointments, while inpatients clustered by the kiosk, buying soft drinks and coffee.

At home I'd been free: free from schedules, nurses, appointments, the constant presence of strangers. I headed toward the elevators, struck by a pang, an aching feeling of being caught between two worlds. I wanted to be independent, to live on my own, but I wasn't quite ready.

Just one more month. One more month and then I'd be free. I'd been transferred to Ward C, the independent ward, where I'd take care of myself, but could still get help if I needed it. It was another step forward.

The elevators opened at the second floor. I veered sharply to the right and took the long way to Ward C. I wanted to avoid passing the nursing station of my previous ward, Ward B.

The day I'd left to go home, I'd given Martha Christmas presents: the latest Danielle Steel novel and a large box of chocolates.

"I hope you have a nice holiday," I'd said after Martha had unwrapped the gifts. "Thank you for everything."

"You've done really well." She smiled gently. "Thank you so much." She held up the chocolates. "My daughter will get into these in no time. We both love them. Now you take good care of yourself."

"You too." And then the intimacy of the last four months was over, just like that.

My life had depended on Martha and now we were practically strangers. She'd probably already been assigned a new "para" or "quad." Accidents, injuries, disease could be counted on. The beds would always be filled.

But I didn't want to stop at the Ward B nursing desk. I didn't want to see anyone I knew. Not even Martha. I wanted a clean break. To move on.

At the Ward C desk, a nurse sorted papers and quietly hummed the "Wind Beneath My Wings." She was in her early thirties, her highlighted blond hair tied back with a pink scrunchie that perfectly matched her frosted nails and lips.

"I'm Susan Mockler." I sidled up to the nursing station. "I'm assigned to this ward now."

"Yes, dear." The nurse consulted a list. "Here you are. We were expecting you yesterday." She frowned: a pouty frown.

"I called to say I'd be coming today instead."

"No record of it, dear. Oh well, you're here now, aren't you?" She forced a tight smile. "I'll show you to your room. *Ooooh.* Aren't *you* lucky? A private room."

236

I was so grateful for Daniel's insurance. It was bad enough to be back here. It would be unbearable to have to share a room.

"By the way, I'm Sandi. With an *I*." She ushered me down the hall. "Wow," she said, when we entered my room. "Looks like you're all set up in here."

"My mom did it yesterday." My clothes, a small TV, a CD player, a few CDs, and some magazines and books were neatly arranged in the room. Enough, I figured, to sustain me for a month. I'd asked my mother to take everything else home, I only wanted the essentials. Tomorrow, my mom was returning to London for the rest of the month and would come back to Ottawa to stay with me the first week after my discharge. Things were moving closer and closer to me being on my own.

"Let's see here," Sandi scanned a sheet. "You only need help getting your meals. Is that right?"

"Yes." Even though I'd made simple meals at home, here everything was served cafeteria-style. With one hand, I couldn't lift plates of food or carry a tray, so I did need help.

"Dressing, bathing, self-care, you're all set?"

"Yes."

"Even your hair?"

"My hair?"

"Your hair is so long. Are you sure you can wash it with just one hand?"

"I've been doing it for more than a month."

"That's good." She nodded. "But you know, dear, you might make it easier on yourself if you cut it. Have you thought of that?"

"I've never had short hair."

"It's a bit different now though, isn't it?"

I didn't answer.

"Well, you can always get a hand, if you need it. All righty, here's your schedule." She handed me a piece of paper. "Any questions?"

"It's pretty clear."

"I noticed you're due in physio in about an hour. Did you see that?"

"Yes."

"Then I'll leave you to it. Remember I'm here if you need anything."

I didn't want to need her. I didn't want to need anyone. I hated having to ask for help. But I had no choice, there were things I couldn't do on my own. Though I didn't want to admit it, I knew this was my new reality, my new life. And it was hard not to resent it, not to feel denigrated by this need, this continued dependence.

But what I didn't have to accept, what I didn't have to get used to, was this affront. What right did Sandi have to question what I could do for myself? To suggest that I cut my hair? To presume she knew better than I did what my capabilities were, what preference I had for the length of my hair? To make me question for just a moment what I knew about my own body? I looked down at my arms. The right was still too spastic to be of any use, but the left was the one I counted on. To go from no arms to one arm and hand was a gift. Martha had helped me see that, had taught me to wash, to dress, to do almost everything one-handed. And I could do these things on my own. I knew that to be true.

About forty minutes later, I left for physio. In the corridor, an elderly man scuffled along then stopped right in front of me, blocking my path. He was tall and stooped. A cheap navy tracksuit spattered with food stains hung off his bony frame.

"Hello there," he said with a strong Ottawa Valley twang. "You're new here, ain't you?"

"I just transferred from Ward B."

"Welcome." He gave me a gummy grin and yet somehow kept hold of the unlit cigarette in one corner of his mouth. "Name's Denny. I've been here going on two months. Couple weeks in intensive care before that. Something burst open in my head. I was just drinking me cup of tea and *bam*. Everything went dark. I'm some better now and they're talking about sending me home. But I ain't ready. Still too weak."

"That's too bad."

"Suppose so." He rubbed his gray bristly chin with one hand. "Of course, we have some fun here. Me and the other men. Play cards every night. Shoot the breeze. And the cafeteria food's real good. Don't you think?"

Another man in a wheelchair dodged around us, nodding curtly as he passed.

"That's Carl. He's heading for a smoke. I better catch up. I've been looking all over for a light."

■ ■ ■

"Today," Sheila said, pointing to a solid wooden frame consisting of four steps, "I thought we'd try stairs. You game?"

"Of course." I rose from my chair. "Do I need my cane?"

"It'll be easier if you use the railing to start."

I moved to the bottom of the stairs. For very short distances, I could balance well enough to stand and step without the cane. Free. I felt so free. "What do I do?" I grasped the wooden handrail with my left hand and peered up the staircase.

"Put your left foot on the first stair then bring your right up beside it. I'll be behind to spot you."

Carefully, I lifted and placed my left, then my right foot, on the step. "There."

"Ready to try the next one?"

"Sure." I leaned heavily on my left arm. My right foot shook slightly but cleared the next step.

At the top of the stairs, the platform was about three feet wide and maybe four feet high, but I felt like I was perched on a high wire. "What do I do now?"

"You'll have to let go briefly to turn around, then grab the railing on the other side. Don't worry, I'm right here."

"Just give me a sec." I felt a little wobbly. My heart thumped. My legs stiffened. I looked down and had a vision of falling, the thwack of my head on the hard tile floor, blood trickling from my mouth, blank eyes. Done. Finally destroyed.

Stop. I could do this.

"You okay?"

"Yes." I inhaled deeply.

"I'll put my hands right here." She extended her arms to either side of my waist, not touching, but ready to catch me if I lost my balance. "Okay. Now turn."

I released the railing and rotated my body, then seized the railing on the other side.

240

"That's it." She patted my shoulder. "Now, to go down, you start by dropping your right foot on the stair, then your left. The opposite of how you climbed up."

Step by step, I descended, confident now in my movements. Terrified during those brief seconds when I'd let go with nothing to cling to, this seemed easy by comparison. By the time I reached the floor, though, my legs were shaking. I sank into my chair.

"That was terrific," Sheila said. "You're fearless, you know? Absolutely fearless. Would you like some water?"

"Please." As she walked away, I turned the word over in my mind. *Fearless?* Not really. I'd been scared, but I hadn't protested. When I'd first ridden in the passenger seat of my mother's car before Christmas, I had anticipated destruction at every turn, but then, like now, I'd endured. I hadn't given in.

Before the accident, I'd often been afraid. As a child, I'd been sleepless with worry almost every night: murderers, burglars, dying before dawn. Saliva pooled in my mouth, and I'd be unsure whether or not to swallow. What if I choked? If I stayed overnight at a friend's house, sleep wouldn't come until I'd meticulously planned an escape route in case of a fire. Houses with second stories and apartment buildings filled me with terror. Later, feeling for lumps and bumps, I was certain that cancer would strike me down. In my twenties, sometimes full-fledged panic had set in.

The first time was in a movie theater in the mid-1980s. I was haunted by a campaign ad I'd watched on TV, by Reagan's grim voiceover as a grizzly ambled across the screen: "There's a bear in the woods." I'd laughed when I saw it, at the ridiculous scare tactics. Then suddenly, inexplicably in the middle of *Paris, Texas*, my thoughts returned to it, to the threat of Russia and raced from the bear to the red button to the nuclear explosion. Now. It could happen any second. Now. Now. Now. My mouth was dry, my body rigid, my heart thudded, and I'd struggled for air. Out. I had to get out. "Bathroom," I'd mumbled to Lisa then fled the theater. Relieved once I'd stepped outside, onto the wide expanse of Bloor Street, into the clear, cold, dark November night.

I'd wasted so much time worrying, but until the accident nothing had happened.

When Daniel and I had first moved in together, after I'd finished my undergraduate degree, we'd ask each other silly questions, maybe to prove our love was real and true.

"How much do you love me?" I'd ask and he'd spread his arms wide and grin. "This much. Even more than this much." I'd felt safe and secure. No one had loved me like that before.

"Would you love me if I were in a wheelchair?"

"Of course," he'd say. "Of course, I would."

At twenty-one, this had seemed like a worst-case scenario, one that could even threaten Daniel's love for me; but it wasn't something that I'd ever envisioned happening. Not really.

But it had. And I couldn't have prevented it. Was I fearless? Not fearless, but maybe more accepting now of the things I could and couldn't control.

"How are you feeling?" Sheila handed me a plastic cup of water. Paper cups were still too difficult. With limited sensation in my left hand, I couldn't get the pressure right and I crushed them. Sheila and I had learned this before Christmas, when an entire paper cup of water had exploded on my lap.

"A little tired. But good. Happy I could do the stairs."

She settled down on one of the steps. "Has Dr. Davis had a chance to talk to you since you've been back?"

"No. Why?"

"We had a new admission over the holidays. A woman in her early forties, a high-level quad. Incomplete. We're hoping she can participate in the body-weight support project. Like you did."

"That's good."

"The thing is, she's very depressed. She was a nurse before the injury and ran a small hobby farm with her husband. A bale of hay fell on her head while they were doing chores in the barn."

Endless. The ways of ending up here were endless.

"She's having a hard time getting motivated to do any kind of therapy. Dr. Davis and I wondered if you would talk to her. Sharing your experience might help."

"Sure."

"Her name is Elise. Maybe the two of you could have lunch?"

JANUARY 9

I CHECKED THE CLOCK. Time to go. Sheila had arranged for me to meet Elise in the cafeteria at one o'clock. I'd just finished lunch in my room. I was still self-conscious eating in public, even here, where so many other people had disabilities like me. At the doorway, I scanned the dining area. Women in chairs were easy to spot. Most of the patients were men. A woman fitting Elise's description was at a table by the window.

"Elise?"

"Yes?" Her voice was soft with a hint of a francophone accent. She had short silver hair and a build so diminutive that she seemed engulfed by her power chair. Her face was drawn, her expression blank.

"I'm Susan. Sheila arranged for us to meet today?"

"Of course." She cast her eyes downward.

"It's nice to meet you." I parked across from her.

"They told me about you. Can you really walk?" She extended her hands to her plate on the table, picked up half a sandwich with one hand, and shakily brought it to her mouth. She took a small bite and then dropped the rest of the sandwich back onto the plate.

"I can walk short distances with a cane but I still need a chair for longer ones."

"Oh." Elise pushed the plate away with her other hand. "They say I must eat, but I have no appetite." She shifted her gaze. Her eyes, dark and intense, trained on me. "How did you ever do it? Start to walk again?"

"I'm in the research study they want you to be in; the body-weight support system on the treadmill. I think that helped a lot."

"I have no movement in the legs."

"I didn't either. I was completely paralyzed right after the accident. You can already use your hands. It took me much longer and I still can't use my right as well as you do. It's only been a few weeks since your injury, hasn't it?"

"Almost a month."

"You're just at the beginning. Still in spinal shock. They told you about that?"

"Yes. But see how weak I am? It's true, I can use the arms a bit, but they do so little. And the legs, they hardly move at all."

"You'll get better and better. You're ahead of where I was. It's a good sign."

"What happened to you?"

I shared the details of the accident. I paused after mentioning the moose, now used to the reaction, as if it were the punch line of a joke. But Elise remained impassive.

"I am very sorry for you. Did Sheila tell you what happened to me?"

"She said you had an accident on your farm."

"I can't stop thinking about it. I replay it over and over. I heard something above me, some kind of rustling, and I

245

looked up. A bale of hay crashed down on me. I keep asking myself, 'Why did I have to look up? Why didn't I just move?' Now, I'm finished. Again and again, I think these thoughts. I can't make them stop." Her eyes filled with tears.

"Sometimes I have thoughts like that too. But you have to push them aside for now, focus on working hard. This is a critical time for recovery."

"That was true for you, but for me, who knows?"

"You're already better. Already using both hands."

"It's not enough."

"But it shows that the nerve impulses are getting through. I know it's very slow. When I feel discouraged, I just tell myself, this is the worst I will be. I will only improve from here."

"I suppose." She sighed. "They want me to take antidepressants. I don't like the idea. I was always a happy person before. But…maybe I should. I don't know. What do you think?"

"It's your decision. But I would. They may help you feel better. I don't think they'd make you worse."

"Perhaps you're right. Oh, here is my husband." A distinguished, silver-haired man in his late-forties strode toward us. He bent down and pecked Elise on the cheek. "Jean Paul, this is Susan. The one I told you about. The one who can walk?"

He held out his right hand. "Very pleased to meet you."

I thrust my left hand forward to meet his. He took it, glancing at where my right hand lay in my lap. I flushed. Until the accident, I'd never realized how often people shook hands. I hated the awkwardness. I was never sure what to do.

"This is all you ate?" he said to Elise, indicating her almost untouched sandwich.

"Je n'ai pas faim. I drank some milk."

"That's good, but you must eat also." He brushed bread-crumbs from the front of her T-shirt.

"You see what he must now do for me?" Elise looked at me.

He put his arm around her and whispered in her ear, worry etched in the lines of his face.

"It was nice meeting you both," I said. "I'm really sorry, but I have to go. I have OT."

"Thank you," she said. "I enjoyed our talk. You are such a brave person, while I...." Her hand fluttered. "I am weak."

I didn't know how to respond. I was out of words. "Bye for now."

On my way to the occupational therapy room, I felt depleted. Elise's hopelessness had drained me.

We were so different. "I've always been happy," Elise had said. But I hadn't, I'd been depressed on and off for most of my life. Though not now, not since the accident.

Whenever I wavered, I forced myself to concentrate on recovery. Any sadness about what had happened or doubts about the future, I blocked out. I disconnected and looked forward. Sometimes, it didn't work and the despair, the loss, seeped through. But I eventually shut the feelings down, shoved them away. I was good at doing that.

So, I was grateful. Grateful for what I used to resent: the hurt, the disappointment, the pain. The need to numb myself to get by. My past had shaped me, made me who I was. I knew how to survive.

JANUARY 17

"I THINK IT'S pretty obvious I can't clean the tub." I peered down into it from my wheelchair.

"We have this," Barb held up a long-handled sponge and passed it to me with a flourish.

I swiped at the bottom of the bathtub. "I still can't reach the far side, the corners, or wipe the taps very well."

"Okay." She jotted some notes on her clipboard. "I feel we've covered the bathroom. What do you think, Deb?"

"Let's go to the kitchen." Deb snapped her laptop shut and heaved herself up from where she sat on the closed-lid toilet. She lumbered down the hall. Barb and I trailed behind. The assessment was being conducted in the independent living unit of the rehab center, a small, one-bedroom apartment down the corridor from Ward C where patients could practice life skills, such as cleaning and cooking, before they returned home.

Deb was my rehabilitation consultant, hired by the insurance company. She was a heavyset woman in her forties with closely cropped, curly black hair and large, round, plastic glasses. Until recently, my mother had dealt with her. Now, I did.

At first, Deb had assured us that I'd get enough money from the insurance company to meet my needs and help me live independently for the rest of my life. But over the last month or so, as we were planning my return home and my future life, Deb seemed to be implementing small but perceptible barriers: hesitating about approvals, creating delays in processing expense reimbursements. I was suspicious and wasn't sure I trusted her anymore.

Her insistence on this housekeeping assessment by my OT was one example. After almost two weeks at home, I knew what I could and couldn't do. My injuries were well-documented. Why couldn't we discuss what assistance I needed and complete the forms that way? Why put me through this?

In the kitchen, at Barb's request, I pulled items from the refrigerator, took out dishes and pots from cabinets, turned on the stove, and rinsed dishes in the sink. Sometimes I stayed in my chair; sometimes I stood.

"Let's try some simple cleaning up," Barb said. "Can you wipe the counter?"

I found a cloth near the sink and ran it over the surface of the countertop. "Now, try this." Barb threw a handful of rice on the floor a few feet away from me.

"You expect me to clean that up?" I asked.

"There's a broom and dustpan in that closet." She pointed across the room. "We have to see how you handle spills."

I wheeled to the closet, deliberately scattering rice across the linoleum with my feet. I grabbed the broom from the closet and leaned it against the wall. It slid to the floor. I picked it up, propped it against the wall again, and started hunting for the dustpan. I found the dustpan and placed it on my lap. The broom clattered to the floor. "This is ridiculous. Even if I manage to bring these over there, I won't be able to sweep up the tiny grains of rice."

"We just needed to see you make the effort," Barb said. "That's fine."

"Okay then," Deb said, typing on her keyboard. "In terms of the kitchen, it looks like we're going to have to rearrange your cupboards at home to make sure your dishes and pots and pans are within easy reach."

"My mom and I already did that. We reorganized the kitchen over Christmas."

"I'm sure you did a fine job, but we'll need to take a look. Make sure you're safe." Deb scrolled through her notes. "And you're going to need a microwave. Taking dishes in and out of the oven is too dangerous. Your left arm isn't strong enough."

"Okay." My arm was getting stronger all the time. I might be able to do it, but I didn't say anything. I wanted a microwave.

"Now, as for housekeeping, you'll need someone to do the heavy cleaning, change sheets, that sort of thing. Some help with daily tidying up, grocery shopping. You're going to do your own laundry, right?"

I'd been doing my own laundry since I'd moved to Ward C. I'd told Deb I wanted to keep doing it at home, but the laundry machines were in the basement of the duplex, down rickety old steps. "As long as you get a washer and dryer for my apartment. But I'll need someone to fold and put away my clothes. Also, some help with cutting up vegetables, like broccoli, cauliflower, carrots, and onions."

"What about your one-handed cutting board?" Barb turned to Deb. "Susan made it herself in OT."

"Harry did most of it." I'd spent many tedious hours sanding the wooden slats. Then Harry, the affable hippie who worked as an OT assistant, had glued the pieces together, hammered in nails that stood upright to spear and stabilize food, and drilled a hole through a knife and attached it to the board with a swivel so that it could be moved up and down like a lever to chop with one hand. "It doesn't work very well. It takes forever to cut with it, and it squishes tomatoes."

"Most people find the cutting board very useful," Barb said.

"I don't."

Barb kept suggesting "assistive devices" for "one-handers." Cheaply made plastic gadgets like button hookers, sock aids, and rocker knives that I often found useless. Figuring out how to do things myself was usually more effective.

And my sister had been the one to solve my most difficult dressing challenge. Not Barb. Not even Martha. Over Christmas, Kathryn had offered to help me put on tights for the first time since the accident, to wear under a new red plaid skirt, but I was able to pull them on by myself without too much difficulty.

"The hardest thing for me is my bra," I told Kathryn. "Even a sports bra one size up is hard to pull over my head and wriggle into. I have to tug and tug at it."

"Just do what I do," she said. "Fasten it, then step into it and pull it over your hips."

"Have you always done that?"

"Yes. It's much easier."

And it was. I'd never even thought to do it that way, nor had any of the women who were helping me. I'd told Barb the strategy when I came back to the rehab center in January so she could pass it along to any other one-armed female patients she might work with in the future.

"I'm sure we can get the insurer to add in some house-keeping hours for food prep," Deb said. "I think we're done here. Thanks, Barb. The sooner you can get your report to me the better. Then we'll go from there. Get everything approved so it's in place when Susan goes home."

Deb walked back to my room with me. At the doorway, she hesitated. "Do you have a few minutes?"

"Sure," I said, though really I wanted her to leave so I could have an hour to myself before physio.

She plunked on a chair and set her laptop case and over-stuffed briefcase on the floor. She hunched toward me, her eyebrows knitting together. "You're still serious about moving to Toronto? Going back to school next September?"

"Yes. Why?"

"Just checking. Want to make sure we have a plan in place."

"Is there some sort of problem?"

She rubbed her hands together. "Not really. It's just that the income-replacement benefits you get are based on the salary you were making as a full-time employee at the time of the accident. If you'd been in school, the amount you'd receive would be lower. If your status changes, I'm not sure what the insurance company will do. They may insist you are only enti-tled to the lower benefit."

"How much would that be?"

"I'll have to check. Maybe three or four hundred a month."

"I can't live on that, and I won't be able to work part-time."

"I know."

"But they've already approved my benefits. They agreed I couldn't do my government job—too much traveling, presentations, all the reasons you gave me before."

"That's true."

"So, if I do nothing, I can keep collecting the benefits. But if I return to school and finish my PhD so that I am qualified to work as a psychologist, a job I will be able to do, then they'll reduce my benefits."

"There's that possibility."

"That doesn't make sense."

"I'll make it clear that it's in their best interests as well as yours for you to return to school."

"Their interests?"

"Financially. Don't worry about it now. I just wanted to make sure we were on the same page before I moved forward. Okay?"

Deb shrugged on her jacket and stood to leave. "You know, it may be a good time to start looking for a lawyer. Not just to deal with the insurance company. You'll want to sue the driver for damages and you only have two years to file a claim."

"Sue Gary?"

"You wouldn't be suing him. You'd be suing his insurance company. You're entitled to damages for pain and suffering. All your other benefits, the ones I'm coordinating, come from your own car insurance company. Through no-fault insurance."

"I don't know if I want to sue Gary." Sometimes, I blamed him for the accident and my injuries. Sometimes I was furious that he'd emerged unscathed with nothing more than a few cuts on his face. But at the same time, I believed what I'd been told. That the moose had come out of nowhere. That there really was nothing Gary could have done. And lawyers, lawsuits, courts, who knew what else? It seemed so messy. I wanted my life to be simple, focused only on getting well. I didn't want any more complications. I didn't want to fight for anything else.

"You should at least talk to a lawyer about it. You might be awarded some money. Money you deserve. Money you will need. That's my two cents, anyway." She hoisted her laptop on one shoulder and picked up her briefcase. "I'll be in touch."

Just when everything seemed to be falling into place, there were more problems. Did I really need a lawyer so soon? While I was still in rehab, still trying to recover? Wasn't that enough to deal with for now?

But money I might need? I didn't know what was going to happen, but I might need a lot. I'd always worked going to school; two, sometimes three jobs at a time. I knew that I wouldn't be able to do that anymore. If the insurance company wouldn't support me returning to school full-time, I was going to need money. Maybe I *would* have to sue Gary.

■ ■ ■

About an hour later, on a mat on the hard wooden floor of the gym, I struggled to get up.

"Let's try this," Sheila said. "First kneel, resting your bum on the back of your calves. Straighten your upper body and swing your right leg in front of you. That's it. Now, put the foot on the floor and shift your weight to the ball of your right foot."

"Okay." I placed my left hand on the ground for balance. "Now what?"

"Rock forward a little, rising up through your right foot, then pull your left…."

"Oh no." I tumbled backward. "That's the third time I've fallen."

"You'll get it. We'll just keep practicing."

"It'd be easier if I had something to brace my left hand on, like a chair or a stool."

"I know. But you never know where you might fall. There may not be anything like that to help you. Let's take a short break. I'll be right back."

I sipped some water. After decades of effortlessly rising from the floor, I now faced this deliberate relearning. I found it so difficult, so frustrating. The complexity of movement, every muscle purposely recruited, each sequence planned, then executed. I had to be able to do it to prove I was ready to go home.

On the other side of the gym, Denny sat on a mat on the floor, his matchstick legs outstretched in front of him, shaking his head from side to side. I listened carefully, straining to decipher what he was saying to his physiotherapist.

"It's no use," he said. "I just can't do it. I ain't strong enough yet. I can't get up off this floor. That's all there is to it."

The physiotherapist murmured, placed her hands on his legs, and attempted to guide him into position. Denny walked better than I did and had full use of both his arms. He was a lot older, but if I was capable of relearning this, he was too. He plopped back on the ground and curled into himself. His voice was louder now, a high-pitched whine. "Don't you understand? I just can't do it. I live all alone. It's not safe for me to go home. I'm not ready yet. It's just not safe."

As hard as I was trying to succeed, Denny was trying to fail. He wanted to stay. His room wasn't far from mine, so I often met him in the hall on his way to the smoking lounge, eager for a chat with the other fellows. I imagined his home, maybe a rooming house in a tiny town in the valley, some small, squalid space, lit by a naked bulb, maybe a hotplate for heating canned beans or making a cup of tea, a lumpy cot, and threadbare sheets. Alone, just getting by. Maybe I was wrong, but to prefer this life to his own, it must be pretty bad.

"Ready to give it another go?" Sheila asked.

"Yes." I shifted onto the mat and, movement by movement, followed Sheila's instructions. I transferred my weight to my right foot, then quickly brought up my left leg, steadied myself with my left hand, and with a final push off the floor, I was up! I was up!

"I did it!" Another step closer to home.

JANUARY 22

I SET MY BOOK on the nightstand. I kept rereading sentences, losing my place. My mind was elsewhere. Had been ever since my meeting with Deb last week. I tried to push away my concerns, but they kept rising up. If the insurance company wouldn't support my return to school, what would I do?

I needed to act. Now. I had to get a lawyer, prepare to fight. Sue Gary. Maybe even my own insurance company at some point.

But could I take on more battles? I blinked back tears. I had to contain myself. If I started crying, I was afraid I might never stop.

It was almost eight o'clock. Daniel would be here soon. I'd missed him. He had been out west the last two weeks for work and a visit with his family. My mother was in London, and without Daniel here I felt disconnected from any other life beyond the rehab center. Nobody here really knew me as me.

I ran a brush through my hair. Daniel would have some suggestions about dealing with the insurance company, about suing Gary. If only we were still together and I could pass along these problems to him, like I had with so many others. He had such a strong way of being in the world. He knew how to get things for himself.

I remembered our trip to Portugal just over four years ago. In mid-July, we'd arrived on a sweltering train to a closed-down station on the outskirts of Albufeira. Along with a crowd of beach-eager tourists, we'd tumbled from the cars, stunned to discover we were in the middle of nowhere. Nothing but dirt, some ragged bushes, and an old man with a donkey.

A lone taxi had skidded to a halt in front of the crowd. Daniel marched through the throng of bodies and within seconds waved to me, victorious. Even without knowing a word of Portuguese, he'd secured the cab, then selected two French Canadian girls we'd been chatting with to share our ride into town. Free from responsibility, I could just go along.

I knew he couldn't solve my problems now, but maybe he could advise me how to deal with lawyers and the insurance company, how to get what I needed, how to win.

A few minutes later, boots stamped along the corridor and Daniel burst into the room. "Hello!" He bent down to kiss my cheek, his face ruddy from the cold, his blue eyes flashing.

"Your lips are freezing." I inhaled his crisp, clean scent, tinged with hints of wood smoke and pine. He smelled like winter. "How was your trip?"

"Great. Mom and Dad are good." He whipped off his coat and settled into a chair.

"Did you see your sisters?"

"They're good too."

I'd loved being part of Daniel's large, boisterous family, their holiday get-togethers, feasts of food and drink, playing board games and charades in teams, the laughter and cries of children scrambling around his parents' house, crawling into my lap and calling me "Auntie."

He unzipped a gym bag and removed a video camera. "Everyone was asking about you."

"That's nice."

"I got Mom to lend me her camera. I have some of our old tapes to show you and I thought I could video you too, so you could send them a message, show them how well you're doing."

"I don't—"

"Let's start with the videos. They should show up pretty well on the wall." He fiddled with cartridges and knobs.

"I need to talk to you about something."

"Can't it wait? I really want to show these to you."

"It's really important. The insurance company may not support me when I go back to school."

"What?"

"The rehab consultant told me. It has to do with my loss of earning benefits. If they reclassify me as a student, instead of employed, I only get a few hundred dollars a month." My voice faltered.

"That's absurd. Did you tell her that? Did you tell her it was unacceptable?"

"I told her it would mean I couldn't go back to school. But maybe I could get student loans again. If I have to."

"Who is this person anyway? Tell her you want to talk to her supervisor or the insurance company directly."

"Please don't shout."

"I'm not." Then more quietly, "It's just—"

"I have to be careful. She has a lot of influence in determining what I get. I need to keep her on my side."

"You still have to stand up for yourself."

"I know…but it's complicated. She told me I should get a lawyer. To sue the driver for damages. That I was entitled to money for pain and suffering."

"That sounds more like it."

"I have to get a lawyer pretty soon. I only have two years to file a claim to sue the driver. And maybe I'll need one to deal with my insurance company too. To get the support I need to go back to school. Do you know how I would get one? A really good one?"

"I can ask around. Someone at the office might know a lawyer who does insurance work."

"That would help me a lot." My shoulders dropped; my whole body released. I hadn't realized how tense I'd been, holding everything in. "Do you want to put on the video now?"

Daniel grinned. "I think you'll really like it." He turned off the overhead lights and flipped a switch on the camera.

Images flashed on the wall: me, Daniel, my mother, grandmother, and sister. My mother's house at Christmas, maybe three years ago. The volume was on, but I wasn't listening, transfixed by this former version of myself, sitting cross-legged on the living room floor, tugging a thread from my jacket sleeve, pushing strands of hair behind my ear: my right ear, my right hand. I was watching a stranger: the fluidity and ease of my movements, the sense of innocence, the unknowing. This was me, before everything fell apart, before everything went wrong. Me, but not *me*.

"Daniel." My throat constricted. "I can't watch this. Can you turn it off?"

"Why?"

"Just turn it off. Right now." I wheeled to the light switch, and flipped it on, obliterating the pictures still flickering on the wall with a harsh, bright, fluorescent glow. Tears welled in the corner of my eyes.

"It's off." He turned to me. "What's wrong?"

"I…." I couldn't speak. I took a deep breath, then exhaled slowly, a shuddering rasping noise, almost a moan.

"Are you okay?"

"It's too hard to watch."

"I'm sorry." He knelt beside me and took my hand. "I thought it would make you happy, bring back good memories."

"I'm just…so different now. I don't want to see. It's not me anymore." I swallowed hard, stifling a sob. I wouldn't, couldn't cry.

"You're still the same person."

"I'm not."

"I know you have these problems, but you're getting better all the time. Look how far you've come."

"I just want to go to bed. Okay?"

"Sure." He gathered his things. "Can I get you anything before I go? Something from the vending machines? Some water?"

"I'm fine. Just tired. I'll talk to you tomorrow."

After he left, I transferred to my bed. The past haunted me. I no longer had any good memories. All I had left was this excruciating sense of loss. I turned on my side and cradled a pillow in my arm. I nestled my face into its soft folds and wept and wept.

■ ■ ■

A wall of black water rose from the ocean. A monster creeping forward, slowly, steadily. Among the shouts and the shrieks, the shoving of the fleeing crowd, I raced to higher and higher ground. Checking over my shoulder, the wave mounted, fifty, sixty feet. I scrambled up, up, up. Its energy thrusted against me, threatening to overtake me, to crush me. I kept running, running, running....

"Help!" A scream. My scream. My sweat-drenched pillow, my hammering heart. I blinked awake.

I sat up, reached for the cup on the nightstand, and sipped some water. I'd had this nightmare three nights in a row.

It was only a dream. The terror. The imminent death. Only a dream.

But only in my dreams was I still swift and strong. Only in my dreams could I feel the wind whipping my hair, my feet thudding along gravel roads, my arms pumping as I sped along, faster and faster. Only in my dreams was my body still free.

"Ready to go for breakfast?" A nurse stuck her head in the door.

"*What?* Um...breakfast? Can you come back in fifteen minutes? I'll be ready then."

■ ■ ■

Later that afternoon, I was in the workout room with Kyle.

"I hear you're going home soon." He handed me a five-pound weight.

"Next week. But I'll still be coming back here three times a week as an outpatient."

"You can't bear to leave all this behind?"

"Not yet."

"You've done great here and you'll do great out there too. It's a big change, but you're ready for it."

"I hope so. You know I haven't seen Jack around lately. Did he get discharged?"

"Just after Christmas. Medically, he was ready to leave before that, but he had nowhere to go. So, they kept him until an accessible unit opened in social housing. He left right away, to scoop it up."

"I wonder what he'll do now?"

"Who knows? We actually went to school together, back in the day. Grades one, two, and three, and then he vanished. Even then, he was always in trouble, picking fights with other little kids, mouthing off to the teacher. And his family was rough. We were all terrified just to walk by his house. You'd go a couple of blocks out of your way to avoid it. They lived right across from the bus station and their front yard was always full of motorcycles and Dobermans, chained up and growling. I think his dad was in the Hell's Angels. Or something like that."

"That's awful."

"It's pretty sad," Kyle said.

"Once he showed me a scar from when he got shot. I was a little scared of him."

"He talked the talk, you know, wanted to be the big,

tough guy, but I think he was more into small-time crime—kind of a low-level dealer, maybe some B and Es, stuff like that."

I had suspected as much. But Jack had been kind to me, and I'd felt a connection and closeness with him that I didn't have with my family and friends. We shared the unexpected tragedy, the sudden loss, and the permanent damage. No matter how much anyone tried, unless they'd experienced it, they couldn't really relate. A gap had been created that couldn't be breached.

Kyle set up the foot cycle and fastened my feet in the straps. He set the timer for twenty minutes. "Be back in a bit." He crossed the room to assist two young guys in chairs.

I started to pedal. I'd tested kids like Jack during my psychology internships. They were usually pale and scruffy, with greasy hair and ill-fitting clothes, and often had behavior problems and learning disabilities. They were the kids whose parents were difficult to contact, even to give them the results of their children's assessments. The odds seemed to be against them right from the start. So what had happened to Jack wasn't all that surprising: a life of petty crime, a bullet wound, a drunken collision with his motorcycle and a wall.

But if an accident had been Jack's destiny, had it also been mine?

Sometimes I felt that my hold on life had always been tenuous. A broken condom was responsible for my conception; an abortion averted largely due to the laws and risks at the time. My mother's slurred complaints: "It was impossible to get an abortion in the 1960s. It was dangerous and illegal. Almost no one could get one." But somehow, my mother's best friend had obtained one in 1965, a year after I was born. "I don't know how she did it, but she was in Toronto. Maybe it was easier there."

Even at fifteen, I understood her message. Sober, she would never have said it, but drunk, she exposed her anger, her wish to have obliterated me. She left other words unsaid, but they echoed in my ears. I'd ruined her life. I'd prevented her from pursuing a master's degree. I'd forced her to marry a man she barely knew who was abusive and later abandoned her. I was to blame.

As a teenager I'd walked the streets of north London almost every night, desperate to escape my life at home. Wandering along the tree-lined streets, I'd felt an overwhelming emptiness when I peered in windows of stately brick houses, the warm glowing lights from dining and living rooms where families gathered, laughing and chatting. Was this how other families were? Was this what a family was supposed to be?

Maybe it was part of my destiny then that after the accident, I would return to this life as I'd started, against all odds, but once again, struggling to survive.

I startled when the timer buzzed.

"Be right there," Kyle called. He released my feet from the pedals. "We were just talking about the Alanis Morissette CD, *Jagged Little Pill*. Have you heard it?"

"Alanis Morissette? The teen pop singer from Ottawa?"

"She's this angry rock chick now. Her album is topping all the charts."

"Is it any good?"

"It's great. Pretty shocking actually. A few of the songs are really explicit. Some radio stations won't even play them."

He pulled the foot cycle from under my wheelchair. "Are you going to walking class now?"

"Yeah."

Kyle glanced into the gym. "It's pretty busy, but if the crowd thins out, I've got the CD. I'll bring in the boom box and play it for you."

I wheeled to the gym. From four to five every day, it was reserved for "walking class," when patients could practice walking the thirty-meter length of the gym. A few chairs were set up in the middle; others lined each side to provide rest points. Each day I tried to go further, increasing the number of laps I walked and reducing how long I rested in between.

I parked at one end. My legs were a little tired from the foot cycle. I'd wait a few minutes before getting started. I sipped water and watched the other patients: some were familiar; others were not.

A tall, lean, Eastern European man sauntered around the gym beside his wife. He nodded to me as he passed. I waved. He was three weeks back in the world after a two-month-long coma. His body was functioning well. He stood erect and proud. But I wasn't sure about his mind. His wife did all the talking.

A man with a lower leg amputation was learning to walk with a prosthesis. Several elderly men and women tread warily, some using canes, others walkers.

My people. For the last six months these had been my peers. I felt safe here. Everyone had experienced illness or injury. Everyone was trying to recover from loss. Was I really ready to rejoin the outside world? It was a world I no longer knew. A world I had to navigate in my damaged body. What would it be like? How would I ever belong?

I took up my cane and joined the procession. Today, I'd walk for thirty minutes, stopping for five-minute breaks every ten minutes. The further I could walk when I left the rehab center, the easier it might be.

As I was nearing the end of my laps, Kyle hurried into the gym, holding up a music player. "Still want to hear Alanis? It's pretty much cleared out in here. I don't think those two will mind hearing a few tunes." He nodded toward two women walking on the far side of the gym, both focused only on their own efforts to move forward. "This song is my favorite." He inserted the CD. "It's called 'You Oughta Know.'"

Softly, almost sweetly, the song began, then the tone and instrumentation shifted, became insistent, unforgiving. As the music pounded through the gym and the rage in Alanis's voice and the frankly sexual lyrics unfurled, I giggled. Across the room, the two women continued on, oblivious to the fury, sex, and betrayal that echoed off the walls. I laughed with pleasure. I laughed with relief. I gasped for air, tears streamed down my cheeks. I laughed: a full, throaty, bodily laugh. The kind of laugh I thought I'd never laugh again.

FEBRUARY 5

"HE'S HERE," I said. The accessible bus rumbled into the driveway. "I'm going now."

My mother came up behind me and adjusted the knapsack that was hanging from the back of my wheelchair.

"Good luck today." She moved to open the apartment door.

"Don't. I have to do everything myself. You won't be here to help me next week."

She backed away and I propelled toward the door, but as I leaned forward to grasp the knob, my wheelchair slid backward and out from under me. I thudded to the floor. "*Shit*. I forgot the brake. Help me up. *Now*. He might leave."

"I'm sure he'll wait. I'll just let him know."

The icy air blasted in as my mom popped outside. "She'll be right there," she shouted to the driver. "Just having a little trouble. Won't be a minute."

I struggled to get up on one knee, then the other. I steadied myself with my left hand on the floor. Perspiration streamed down my face. It was almost impossible to move swaddled in my down parka and snow boots. I lifted my right knee then tumbled back on my bum. Not again! Forcing my right side from the ground was like raising half a corpse. Maybe I couldn't do this. Maybe it was all too much.

"He'll wait," my mother said, quickly shutting the door.

I wouldn't give up. I'd made it this far.

"Just give me your arm, would you, Mom?" I braced against her, stood up, and settled back in my wheelchair. "Why did you tell him that I was having trouble? He didn't need to know that."

"I don't know." She looked a little hurt. "I guess I thought he'd be sympathetic."

"To a crippled girl who can't even get herself out of her own apartment."

"*What?* Nobody thinks that. It's your first time going to the rehab center on your own. There's bound to be little mishaps. Don't worry. Everything will be fine."

"I'm not worried. I've just got to go."

On the porch, I pivoted my chair to lock the outside door. Although my left hand didn't actually feel the cold, my fingers became stiff and clumsy. But I'd practiced this. I removed my left mitten with my teeth, and then inserted the key into the lock. My hand shook. Steady. Be steady. I turned the key. *Click.* The bolt slid into place.

I made my way down the stair lift and onto the driveway. I extended my left leg to kick forward and move toward the bus, but the driver scooted over.

"Let me give you a hand there, Miss," he said, each word a puff of frozen droplets in the air. He grabbed the back handles of my chair and wheeled me up the ramp into the bus. I wanted to refuse his help, insist I could do it myself, but I was already tired and my day hadn't even begun.

"Thanks. Sorry I was late."

"No problem. You're the only rider on this trip." He adjusted the straps and belts, securing my wheelchair to the floor of the bus.

We chugged down the street, and I started to relax. I removed my toque and placed it in my lap and smoothed my sweat-drenched hair. Today was already such an ordeal. But I was on my way now. Each day would get better. And I wouldn't let myself fall out of my wheelchair again!

"Have a good day," the driver said, when we reached the front doors of the rehab center.

I entered the foyer with a dislocated sense of familiarity, like returning to high school a few years after graduation. The environment was intimately known, but something was different: I no longer quite belonged. I wheeled to a quiet corner to remove my outdoor clothing.

Overclothes now piled in my lap, I checked the clock on the wall. About fifteen minutes until my first appointment. A young woman in a power chair accompanied by an attendant approached the reception area just a few feet away. She must be a high-level quad. I couldn't detect any movement in her arms, nor did she have a "sip and puff" mechanism that would allow her to use her breath to drive her chair. The attendant tugged off the woman's wool hat to reveal a strap across her forehead securing her to the headrest and a metal device pressed against her cheek. Was that how she controlled her chair?

"Next," the clerk called, and the two women moved to the reception desk. I couldn't hear his question, but after the clerk had spoken, the attendant turned to the woman in the chair. "One, two, three, four," she said. "One two, three, four, five, six…."

Curious, I edged closer.

The woman in the chair blinked in response to the number "six." She was communicating by blinking her eyes! Locked-in syndrome. That must be what she had. I'd heard about it from one of the nurses: every part of the body was paralyzed except the eyes, yet the person was fully conscious and cognitively intact. Not able to talk or sign, their only means of expression was through eye movements.

Less than an hour ago I'd been filled with despair, thrashing about, trying to get up from the floor by myself. The shame of it now. Independence didn't necessarily mean doing something completely on your own. Just like this woman, I needed assistance to do things and be out in the world. I still wanted to do as much as possible myself, but receiving help didn't diminish or devalue me or anyone else who needed it. That's just how it was. And that was okay.

■ ■ ■

Several hours later, after physiotherapy and walking in the gym, I headed to the lobby to eat the lunch I'd prepared and packed last night: an apple, a few pieces of cheese, crackers, and baby carrots. Simple, but nutritious. I wheeled to the snack kiosk.

"I'll have an orange juice, please." I laid a five-dollar bill on the counter. This was the first time I'd purchased something since the accident.

"That's two dollars." The clerk handed me the juice. I nestled the bottle in the open knapsack on my lap and raised my left arm to take the change. I couldn't feel the three loonies in my hand, but I kept my eyes there, grasped the dollar coins tightly in my fist, and dropped them in my bag. So far, so good.

I parked by a window. Outside, the bright sun glinted on the snow. I fished out the bottle of juice. A screw-top lid. Hmm. I wedged the knapsack between my left thigh and the arm of the chair to give me room. I stabilized the bottle between my knees and twisted the cap hard. It didn't open. Again, I gripped and turned with as much strength as I could. *Pop!* The lid released.

I looked around the room at the others in chairs or with canes or walkers. No one was familiar. Most of the patients I knew had probably been discharged. That morning in physio, I'd learned that the injured nurse, Elise, had already gone home, was finished with rehab altogether.

"So soon?" I asked.

"She was medically stable, and we couldn't do much more for her," Sheila had said. "She stopped participating in the body-weight support research and wasn't making any further progress."

"That's too bad."

"She'll be happier there. Luckily, their farmhouse was fairly accessible. They didn't have to do many renovations."

After our lunch, I'd only seen Elise a couple of times when we passed in the halls. Elise still used a power chair, always accompanied by her husband. Her expression was sad as she smiled wanly and nodded. She had shown such promise, her initial recovery better than mine. But while Elise's gains had stopped, I'd continued to improve, was still improving now. Why? Was it the differences in our injuries? How we'd coped? Or maybe it was just random, out of our control.

Although sometimes I flirted with ideas about fate and destiny and whether there was an underlying meaning, a reason behind my accident, what I'd really come to believe was that life was random. That the things I'd been born with and the things that had happened to me were largely out of my control. There were things I could change and things I couldn't change. Things that I needed to let go. All I could do was work as hard as I could within my own limits. And that if I focused on that most of the time, I'd probably be okay. Maxims so simple they could be bumper stickers and yet I now knew them to be true.

Outside, I glimpsed the two women of the trio in rose-colored parkas with matching pink-and-white striped toques, stamping along the snow-covered path. But where was the man? Had something happened to him? No, there he was, just a few feet behind, in a navy parka and blue-and-white striped hat. When he caught up to the women, all three paused. He extended his gloved hands, presenting each of them with a glistening snowball. Exquisitely sculpted: two perfect spheres.

For over half a year, I'd observed this trio. At first, completely paralyzed in my bed, the halo drilled into my skull, logrolled on my side by the nurses, through a dust-streaked window, under a late August sun. Then from my power chair, parked in a garden on the hospital grounds, among the whispers of falling red and yellow leaves. And now, here they were again on my first day as an outpatient. In a way, they'd become touchstones of this new life.

I unlocked the brakes on my chair and dropped my apple core and juice bottle in the garbage. Time for OT, and then my first day was over.

In the occupational therapy room, I wheeled to the shelf where my basket was stored. When Barb had suggested basket weaving as therapy for my left hand, I'd thought she was joking.

"Seriously?" I asked. "Basket weaving?"

"It can be helpful for promoting fine motor skills and working in the water also stimulates sensation," Barb said. "Besides, it's an independent activity."

I reached into my cubby marked by a piece of masking tape where I'd scrawled my name with my left hand. I dumped my basket into my lap and grabbed a handful of reeds from the supply area. I moved to the sink and plunked the basket and reeds in the basin. I rose to my feet, fumbled to put the stopper in place, ran the water, and waited for the level to rise high enough to soak everything. I turned off the tap, sat back in my chair, and poked at a few of the reeds with a long wooden spoon. I wanted to be on the computer or practicing writing with my left hand, but Barb had been adamant, twenty minutes of basket weaving before each of our sessions.

It was like home economics all over again. Mrs. Hollis, my Grade 8 teacher, brandishing a knitted pink bunny and an orange-and-yellow scarf at the front of the room. "Well done, girls," she'd said, beckoning her two favorite students forward to reclaim their prized efforts. "Outstanding. This is what everybody should be aiming for." I'd been called last, as the parade of triumph turned to one of failure. "Really, *black*?" Mrs. Hollis scowled as she returned my lumpy attempt at a pincushion, purportedly the easiest of the knitting projects, a grading slip with a big, fat, red *D* affixed to it. "At least you could have picked a cheerier color."

Who cared? I stood again, picked up a reed, and listlessly tried to thread it through the strands that protruded from the basket's base.

After what seemed like forever, Barb tapped my shoulder. "Ready for our session?"

"Yes." Thankfully, this was over.

Barb plucked the basket from the water. "Nice job. But… well…you don't seem to be getting very far with it. Put your things away and meet me over there." Barb pointed to a table across the room. "And park your chair. I'd like to see how your walking is coming along."

I walked to the table. I still leaned heavily on my four-pronged cane, but my speed and stride length were improving. I took a seat at the table.

"Your walking is really progressing. Your hard work is definitely paying off." Barb took my right arm and began range of motion stretches.

I closed my eyes and concentrated on relaxing the spasticity in the arm, hoping that this would make the stretches more effective.

When I opened my eyes again, Eddie, a relatively new admission, strolled into the room. He was swinging a straight cane, a cardboard box tucked under his arm. In his early twenties, over six feet in height, his fit build was still evident, despite the spinal injury he'd suffered after being slammed into the boards during an intramural hockey game. He stopped at each table, his mop of red hair bobbing, chatting with each therapist and patient in turn.

I'd heard about him a week or so before we'd met. One day, working out with Kyle in the exercise room, a few of the male patients were chattering about him.

"You wouldn't believe this guy," his roommate had said. "First day. Gets right out of bed. Walks to the bathroom and takes a leak. All by himself."

"Holy shit!" another one said. They all nodded in amazement as if they'd heard an eyewitness account of Clark Kent transforming into Superman.

I knew how they felt. How was it even possible? And as with the teenaged girl who'd been here in the fall and seemed to recover within a week, I was jealous.

Last week Eddie and I were introduced for the first time during a joint OT appointment with Barb, who was demonstrating a toenail clipper bolted to a piece of wood that supposedly could be used as an aid to safely cut nails with one hand. Like me, Eddie couldn't use his right hand.

"Barb tells me we have the same injury," Eddie had said.

"Really?" I hoped the dismay didn't show on my face.

"Susan's injury is more severe, Eddie," Barb had said.

"But you're improving too, aren't you?" he'd asked.

"Sure." I'd thought of Jack's words: "Why do some people get so much better and others don't?"

"Susan's progress has been incredible," Barb had said. "Absolutely remarkable."

When Eddie reached our table, he pulled out a chair to

join us. "Care for a doughnut, ladies?" He set the box down and grabbed a seat. "I would've brought coffees, but I can only carry so much with the cane in my good hand. You know what I mean." He winked at me.

I was impressed by the way he'd clutched the box under his right arm. Maybe I could do that too. I bit into the sugary doughnut. "Thanks."

"I saw you walking in the gym today. Booting along. You looked great."

"You too. Your walking is excellent. You're barely using your cane."

"Still, the hand." He held up his right. "But yeah, I'm doing good. They're discharging me next week. I'll be an out-patient. Like you."

"That's great." Like me? Not quite.

"You aren't finished here with Barb yet, are you?"

"No." I looked at her. "Not for a few more minutes, right?"

"Be back in a sec." Cane tapping, Eddie sauntered toward the woodworking shop.

"What's going on?"

Barb smiled. "We'll have to wait and see."

When Eddie returned, he placed a tissue-wrapped object in front of me. "For you." A wide grin spread across his liberally freckled face.

"Wha—?" I tugged away the paper to reveal a masterfully crafted, one-handed toenail clipper. Eddie had shellacked a rectangular piece of wood about six inches long and two inches wide. He'd bolted the nail clippers at one end and carved the other into the shape of a heart with my initials

burned in the center, etched in elaborate calligraphy. "Thank
you so much. You did an amazing job."

"Harry helped me a lot, especially with the design and the
letters. I made myself one too. Not as fancy."

"It's the perfect gift for me."

"Glad you like it. Just hope you won't always need to use
it, you know?"

"I do." My voice caught in my throat.

■ ■ ■

"How did it go?" My mother flew to the door as I wheeled
inside, freezing, after a chilly ride on the accessible bus. I felt
like I was returning from my first day of school.

"Pretty well." I fought to remove my coat. My mom
moved to assist me, then took a step back.

"I'd like your help. I'm exhausted."

"Once you get used to the routine, you won't be so tired."

"I hope not."

"I was going to start dinner but wasn't sure if you wanted
me to. If you wanted to do it yourself?"

"No! I'm going to take a nap. Maybe when I'm at therapy
this week, you could cook some meals to freeze, then when
I'm on my own I can just reheat them in the microwave if I'm
tired?"

"I'd love to do that for you, honey."

"And Mom…I'm sorry I yelled at you this morning. I
think I was really anxious."

"I understand. I was nervous too." She hugged me tightly,
and for once I didn't resist, I didn't pull away.

FEBRUARY 26

FROM THE DOCK, my grandparents' cottage looked the same—red wooden slats, white gingerbread trim, small but cozy. A loon called. I inhaled the deeply familiar pine-scented air. My right foot dragged along the uneven terrain: pitted limestone, clumps of moss. The door was unlocked. I swung it open and went inside. Coughed. Sneezed. Everything was cloaked in thick dust. Spider webs curtained the corners, the doorways. Preserved, but deserted. Had no one been here in the last twenty years?

In the room I'd shared with my parents as a child during the summers, cupboards lined the walls. I opened the first one. Photographs spilled out. Black-and-white shots of my grandparents' wedding, my mother in a poodle skirt and bobby socks. A baby—me—in a long, lacy christening gown. Polaroids from the early 1970s: me in a purple two-piece driving the small motorboat, Kathryn as a toddler sitting in a plastic pool, my parents in lawn chairs drinking beer on the dock. I placed the photos on the cot where I used to sleep. I was taking these with me.

The next cupboard: my clothes, jewelry, posters, the

contents of my room in first-year university. I selected a pair of silver hoop earrings, a paisley scarf, a print of Picasso's *Blue Nude* that had curled at the edges. A photo of Daniel and me fluttered to the floor. Smiling, arms around each other, on the ferry to the Toronto Islands, Hanlan's Point, tennis rackets at our sides, a bag holding our picnic lunch. Our first summer together.

In a third cupboard, books crammed the shelves: *Fun with Dick and Jane*, *The Bobbsey Twins*, *The Catcher in the Rye*, *To the Lighthouse*, *For Whom the Bell Tolls*, *Fear and Trembling*, *The Waste Land and Other Poems*, *Introduction to Psychology*, Hays's *Statistics*. I paged through the stats book: probability theory, random assignment. Then I saw Annie Proulx on the spine of a paperback tucked in a far corner. I tugged it out. The title had faded away, but I knew it. Had taken it with me on the trip to read in New Hampshire when Gary and I reached the mountains.

I surveyed the pile on the bed. Time to go.

I filled two pillowcases that I stripped from the bed. Heavy, so heavy in my left arm. I tottered forward, stumbled, lost my balance, nearly fell. Too much to carry. I had to choose what to take, what to leave behind. But I wanted it all.

The ringing of the telephone jarred me awake. Phone? Phone? I fumbled under the pillow.

"Hello?" Groggy. Drugged with sleep. Still immersed in the landscape of my dream: my grandparents' cottage.

"Did I wake you up?" Deb, my rehab consultant, asked.

"No. Maybe. What time is it?"

"Around nine."

"I guess I slept in. I don't have rehab today."

"I've got some great news. I've convinced the insurance company to support our plan for you to return to school to finish your PhD."

"Really? With full financial support?"

"They'll review it each year, but I made them understand that if you finish—"

"I'll finish."

"—and become a registered psychologist, you will be able to earn some of your pre-accident income."

"So, it's good for them too."

"Well, yes."

"It *is* good news. I'll have to call York. My advisor. The department. Figure out what to do next."

"Keep me posted. Don't do anything until we've discussed it first."

I leaned on the cane and pulled myself out of bed. Bathroom. Kitchen. Coffee. A little stunned: the vivid dream, Deb's news. I rested the cane against the counter and gingerly carried my coffee to the table, trying to keep my balance, trying not to spill. I was so much freer now that I could take more steps without the cane. Hopefully, soon, I wouldn't need it at all.

My hand shook a little as I sipped my coffee. So much to plan. So much to do! I should call Daniel. Tell him my news.

I headed to my bedroom to retrieve the cordless phone. It was almost three weeks since my mother had left, and I remained nervous at night. I tried to block images of rapists and burglars prizing the door, shattering the windows, attacking me while I was unable to defend myself, to fight back. In the rehab center, I'd felt safe. Nurses and staff patrolled the halls and immediate help was available by pressing a call bell. But here, I was completely alone.

Twice, the winter before my accident, kids had broken into my apartment. At least, the police had guessed they were kids based on what they'd taken. The first time it was about twenty dollars' worth of change from a coffee tin, half a pack of cigarettes I'd hidden from myself in a drawer, and my sapphire engagement ring with the cracked silver band. The police had provided me with a list of pawn shops so I could search for the ring, but I'd never bothered. Part of me was relieved to no longer possess this reminder of my marriage, this remnant of hope. The second time, the thieves had taken about five dollars in change. They'd left behind the TV, the VCR, and my computer. I didn't have much else.

The break-ins were about a month apart. Both times, they'd climbed onto the air conditioning unit and forced open a living room window, leaving behind oversized sneaker prints in the snow. Both times I'd been out, arriving home to frigid temperatures, papers fluttering through the room driven by the gusts from the open window, drawers and cupboards ajar. I'd notified the police, but hadn't felt much of anything: not violation, not terror, just a mild annoyance, something else unpleasant to deal with. I'd been so numb then. I knew that now. Sleepwalking through each day. Living, but not living. Absent. Not in my life at all.

After the second break-in, the landlord had installed motion detector lights by the windows, and no one had ever returned. It was enough of a deterrent for them to move on, or maybe they realized I really had nothing left.

I'd more or less forgotten about the robberies, but now the

memory of them scared me. I was more alive in my feelings now, more able to experience the fear than when the break-ins had happened. I also felt more vulnerable living alone than I had before my injury. But I refused to let it disrupt what I'd finally achieved: independence, a home of my own.

So, each night before I went to bed, I double-checked the locks on the windows and doors. I slept with the bathroom light on and the cordless phone by my side. That seemed to help.

■ ■ ■

I punched in Daniel's number, then his extension. "Hello," he answered before the second ring.

"Daniel?"

"Hey. How are you?"

"Great. Really great. Guess what? The rehab consultant just called. They're going to support me so I can go back to school."

"That's…terrific."

"It's such a relief. I'm nervous. But mostly I'm excited."

"You're definitely moving to Toronto?"

"Yes."

"When will you go?"

"Maybe August? I'm going to see if I can get student housing. An apartment right on campus would be the easiest for me. I have so much to do."

Silence. Unusual for Daniel and then the full implication of my decision hit me. Despite our separation, we'd remained tethered to each other as close friends, but there was something more. The possibility of reconciliation always hung between us. Daniel had even hinted at it a few times over the year.

"We'll still talk on the phone," I said. "I can see you when you come to Toronto for work." We'd always be friends, I knew that. But my departure meant things were really over.

"I'm happy for you." His voice hoarsened. "But I've got to go. Have to finish a report by the end of the day. I'll call you later." He hung up quickly: a click and then a dial tone in my ear.

I felt a tender sadness as I hung up the phone, but I knew this was the right decision. As much as I loved Daniel, I couldn't live under his expectations and scrutiny, his stifling control. I had to be free to determine my own actions, to discover who I would be in this new life. I went to my desk and pulled open the drawer. My dissertation proposal lay on top, where I'd left it at Christmas. I picked it up and started reading. It was time to return to it now.

FEBRUARY 29

I STOOD BY THE window and waited. The last couple of mornings I'd watched for him, learned his routine. He arrived at nine-thirty, usually on the dot. Today I was prepared, dressed in my winter clothes, ready to hurry outside at the first glimpse. I spied his black boot in mid-stride as he passed the wooden fence separating my house from the neighbors'. I headed out the door.

"Hello." I waved to the lanky, bearded man who had stopped at the end of the driveway. "Can you come over here for a sec?"

"What for?" he grunted as he hoisted his carrier bag on his shoulder.

"I just want to ask you something. I can't come to you." I held up my cane and shook it in the direction of the snow-covered pavement. "It's too slippery."

He yanked his postal cap down over his ears and slogged toward me. "What exactly can I do for you, Miss?" He jutted out his chin.

"I'm so glad to see you. About a month ago, my mailbox was moved from the front of the house to here." With my cane, I waved toward a rectangular black metal box with a gold-colored "2" painted on it, mounted on the wall beside my apartment door. "I got mail for a while, but then it stopped over a week ago. I thought you might be new. Maybe you didn't know?"

"I knew. I tried it for a bit, but it takes up too much time, interferes with my route. Besides, there are union rules. We're not supposed to deliver to more than one location per address. I can't come all the way around the corner down this driveway when there's a perfectly good box for you at the front of the house. That's where I deliver for this address. Always have. Always will. No exceptions."

"But that's the other apartment's front door. I can't go up those stairs anymore. I was in a bad car accident. That's why we moved my box here. My rehab consultant called. The post office said it would be okay."

"You'll have to take it up with them." He spun around.

"Wait! Just wait. Where's my mail? The mail you haven't delivered?"

"That'd be up at the postal station on Riverside. You can go collect it there."

Inside, I put on the kettle. What a jerk! Easier for him to lug my mail back to the postal station than walk ten steps out of his way?

I carried my teacup, half-filled so it wouldn't spill, to the living room, and set it on the coffee table. I picked up the phone to dial Daniel at work, to get his advice, and then hung up. I walked a few steps to the bookshelf and removed the phone book, heavy in my hand, stumbled a little, took a few more steps, and settled on the couch. I hunted through the government blue pages for the number.

After three postal officials, they finally connected me to the correct supervisor.

"That's Alf for you." He chuckled. "He's a bit of a stickler. But not to worry, Miss. Give me a couple of days to straighten things out and we'll have your mail delivered right to your box at the side door."

"Thanks very much." Would Alf be reprimanded? Assigned another route? I hoped so but didn't ask. I'd gotten what I needed.

"If nothing shows up in your box within a few days, call me back. But everything should be okay from here on in. I'm really sorry about the mix-up."

I hung up the phone. I could have been more strident, more outraged as Daniel would have been, but I'd asserted myself in my own way and it had worked. A small victory, but it meant so much.

I returned the phone book to the shelf next to the scrapbook my sister had compiled over the Christmas holidays. Early on, one of the nurses had suggested collecting all the notes, letters, and cards that I received during my time in the hospital as keepsakes to put in a book. "Most patients find it helpful to document this time in their lives," the nurse had said. I wasn't interested. But my mother had kept everything, and Kathryn had filled the blank pages of a leather-bound album. I couldn't look at it then. It was too soon, too close.

But today, I was drawn to it. I placed the scrapbook on my lap and began leafing through the pages. My mother had been meticulous. Everything was here: the hospital bracelet from the neuro-observation unit, cards that had been enclosed with bouquets dating from the second day after my accident, get-well wishes, letters. So many people had reached out. There were other mementos too: a placard of a Bible verse with "I love you" written at the bottom in my grandmother's wobbly hand, the label from the bottle of Lourdes holy water my father had brought on his first visit, a pressed yellow rose from Daniel, scarlet and golden maple leaves that my mom and I had gathered on the wooded path beside the rehab center on our outings in late September. A snapshot of me in the halo, upright on the body-weight support system in early October. Taped to the last page was the front cover of the rehab center's fundraising brochure that I'd agreed to pose for in December. Seated in my wheelchair, I smiled for the camera, my left arm raised in a biceps curl, a five-pound weight in my hand.

Day by day, week by week, month by month, shifting states of body, of mind, of self. Though I wished it wasn't, this was part of me. Of who I was now and who I'd always be.

I placed the scrapbook on the coffee table and a couple of loose papers wafted to the floor. Not part of my mother's collection, but items I had shoved in the back of the album after Kathryn and then my mom had left. I retrieved a square of thin newsprint and for the first time in months, studied the black-and-white image. A dead moose beside a crumpled car and the caption below with my name and the fateful sentence: "Une femme, 31, d'Ottawa était sérieusement blessée." I slid the newspaper clipping into the front of the scrapbook. This really was the first entry, the beginning of my story, the beginning of this new life.

I grabbed the envelope that had also drifted to the floor. Mr. Semple's name and address neatly printed in block letters in the upper left-hand corner, the reminder of the "affair." I'd held onto it since Thanksgiving, not ready to read it, unsure if I'd ever be. But I no longer cared what he'd written, what he wanted from me. I wasn't a victim. He had no hold on me.

In the kitchen, I tossed the letter in the garbage along with the other scraps from my morning: two sodden tea bags, an empty yogurt container, and a banana skin. I closed the lid of the bin. Done.

■ ■ ■

By late-morning, the maintenance crew had shoveled the driveway, the sky was cobalt, the snowbanks sparkled, and the outdoors beckoned. I decided to take a walk outside. On my own for the first time. I was ready. I could do it.

My right leg tremored as I descended in the stair lift, but I stepped onto the driveway and weighted my right foot, quieting the spasm. One foot then the next, transferring from right to left, left to right, step by step, I made my way to the sidewalk. My first instinct was to turn left, toward the canal. On weekday mornings, the speed skaters took to the ice. In winters past, if I had a day off, I used to run along the canal, hoping my timing would coincide with their practice. With their smooth movements, their effortless gliding, singly or in pairs, they seemed to float, hovering over the surface, a perfect unity of body and motion. Even before the accident, I hadn't been able to skate like that. But today, I didn't want to observe such physical grace as I limped along.

I veered right, toward Bank Street. If I could manage a block and a half, I could stop for a coffee. I'd envied Kathryn over the holidays, casually going out to grab a coffee. Yet just over a month later, here I was, out of the house, on my own. I edged forward, eyes trained on the ground, left hand clenching the cane, focusing on each step. The sidewalk was icy, jagged. Ruts formed from prior thaws now refrozen, some random, but others discernable, vestiges of movement, like archeological remains of previous passersby: the shape of a child's boot, sled tracks, the paws of a dog, the deeper, larger, rounded imprints of an adult who'd worn mukluks.

Halfway down the block, I paused to rest. I was alone on the street. Bare branches of trees extended skyward; an off-leash black Lab scampered across a lawn. Everything was so familiar yet different and new. I swung my cane forward. Right foot. Left foot. One. Two. Step. Step. On Bank Street, the sidewalk was less treacherous, scraped clear to the pavement by shopkeepers and restaurant owners.

The sign for the café was just a half-block away.

Ahead of me, two women about my age in running gear were walking briskly, probably cooling down after a jog. The cadence of their steps, as they flowed along, their arms swinging, every joint working together, effortlessly, burned into me. Seven months ago, that had been me, and now this arduous struggle just to creep forward. I wanted to turn around, skip the café, and drag myself home. But no. This was how it was going to be out in the world. I had to face it, or I'd trap myself forever, hidden away in a room. And that was not how I wanted to live.

At the café, I tilted my cane against the wall and pried

open the door. Its cumbersome weight, the small step at the entryway, obstacles that of course I'd never noticed before. But I made it. I was in!

I trudged to the counter, my legs heavy with fatigue. "A skim milk latte, please."

"Right." The young woman glanced up from a magazine. "I know you. You used to come in here all the time. I thought you'd moved."

"No," I flushed, feeling her eyes on me, taking me in. But I was here now, I couldn't—wouldn't—care. "Car accident."

"What a sin. Are you going to be okay?"

"I'll be fine."

"Take a seat and I'll bring your coffee right over. Do you want cinnamon or chocolate sprinkles?"

"Cinnamon, please. Thanks."

I chose a table by the window, large glass panes giving me a full view of the street. "Here you go." The server set down my drink.

Across the road, a mother pulled a toddler on a red toboggan, a clutch of school children were laughing and running together, an elderly woman determinedly pushed a bundle buggy full of groceries along the street. I smiled, immersed in the pleasure of sipping my latte as I witnessed and felt part of the life around me.

Over the last seven months, part of my survival, my recovery, had depended on my ability to push thoughts and feelings away, to continue on despite fear and loss, always looking forward, hoping for more. Here, now, in this quiet, ordinary, yet extraordinary moment, out in the world again, I could let everything in.

I was tired on the way home, but I walked with more confidence. I still kept my eyes down, scanned the path ahead for patches of black ice or lumpy ridges of snow. I didn't want to fall.

"Whoa there. Watch where you're going."

I looked up. I'd almost collided with a man, maybe in his sixties, dapper in a camel coat and fedora, a green plaid scarf nestled around his neck. "I'm sorr—"

"No. I'm sorry." His voice softened. "I didn't see." He gestured to my cane. "You have a problem with walking?"

"Yes."

"Did you break your leg? Have a skiing accident?"

"Something like that."

"Well, you're young. I'm sure you'll heal up in no time. Take care." He tipped his hat and strode away.

A skiing accident. A broken leg. He'd mistaken me for someone for whom disability was a temporary inconvenience, a transitional state, not a new identity, a radically altered life. A skiing accident. But that could be something more, like it had been for Jill Kinmont from *The Other Side of the Mountain* and for Peter, my colleague from work.

I could walk with a cane and use my left hand. I might improve a little more, I hoped so, but I knew that I would never fully recover.

I had a new body, a new life, new challenges, but also more clarity, more certainty. Things would be hard, but I knew I was going to be okay. I took another step toward home, feeling lighter, as if relieved of a burden, a respite from loss.

EPILOGUE

I chose to end this memoir as I embarked on my new life. That was over twenty-five years ago, when I viewed my recovery as a reclamation of self and was eager to re-enter my life. I had little understanding of what I would experience now that I was disabled. I didn't realize that disabled meant I had crossed an invisible line and become "other" to the world at large and even, in some ways, to myself.

Almost a year after the accident, I moved back to Toronto to attend university full-time and complete my doctorate in psychology. At that time, I no longer used a cane, but because my right leg was spastic, I walked slowly and with a limp. I also had very little function in my right arm.

Though I was open about my disability, needs, and limitations with my family and close friends, I was shy and self-conscious with strangers. Not even fully aware of what I was doing, I now realize I was trying to hide my disability, to pass as "normal."

In university classes, I was quiet and reserved. I avoided contact and remained seated while others left together for a coffee break. At the few parties I attended, I remained still and avoided any movement that would reveal my limitations.

One day, my sister and I were sampling lipsticks at a department store cosmetics kiosk. The salesclerk asked me to sit on a high stool at the counter, one that was impossible for me to perch on. I replied that I preferred to stand. As we left with our purchases, I said, "I don't think she noticed that there was anything wrong with me." In that moment, I was elated to be mistaken for "normal."

In my first years as a clinical psychologist, this desire to appear able-bodied continued. In initial assessments and sessions with clients, I avoided shaking hands because I had to use my left, which might result in a need for me to admit that I couldn't use my right. At the clinic, I arrived first to meetings and left last so I wouldn't have to expose my "awkward" gait. These attempts seldom worked, and ultimately I would explain that I had been in a car accident. When asked if I would get "better," I would respond "maybe," not wanting to disclose that disabled was now my permanent state.

In new situations, whether professional, social, or educational—really any time I was out in the world—I persisted in trying to mask my disability.

I forced myself to adapt to the able-bodied world. I ignored pain and fatigue to my own detriment, injuring myself several times by overdoing it physically. I only sought and accepted help or accommodation when doing something by myself was otherwise impossible.

Then, about ten years ago, I missed a connecting flight, refusing to use the accessible services at the airport, though I walked too slowly to reach the gate in time. As I waited for the next plane, I realized I needed the assistance. I was disabled.

Following this, my attitude gradually shifted. Now, I make no attempt to conceal my disability and I refer to myself as "disabled." It is part of me, as central to the core of myself as any other physical, intellectual, or emotional attribute.

I now know that my internalized ableism underlay my desire to appear "normal." I did not want to be seen as disabled. I was ashamed. I had adopted the socially inculcated views that disabled people were "less:" less capable, less intelligent, less attractive, less worthy. The list of "less" is endless.

While it took over a decade of being disabled to admit my own prejudice, this new understanding helped me to reinterpret my experience. I stopped trying to conform to able-bodied conceptions of how I should be and took notice of how the attitudinal and physical barriers I faced often denigrated and excluded me.

Public scrutiny of my body was initially surprising. In line for coffee, walking along the street, traveling by taxi, people would ask, "Did you have a stroke? An accident? What happened to you?" I felt on display and that I'd lost my right to privacy. I longed to be invisible, to be left alone. People often offered me advice or encouragement as one would to a small child: "Good for you to be out on your own!"

Other intrusions were more hurtful. "What's the matter with you anyway?" a cab driver once asked me after I got into his taxi.

"I was in an accident," I replied.

"You can't use your arm? And you don't walk very well. Christ," he said. "If I was you, I'd kill myself."

Just three years ago, while seated on a bench in a

community center change room, I was putting my T-shirt over my wet bathing suit after a swim, thinking about whether to pick up a sandwich for lunch on the way home. A woman at the next locker, still in conversation with two friends, came over and tugged my shirt on for me. She pulled my less functional arm through the sleeve, without saying a word to me. I was speechless.

Still chattering to her friends, she returned to clothing herself, glancing over at me periodically. Humiliated, I pulled my shorts on halfway. As I bent over to slide my left foot into my shoe, she swooped in, and again without asking, put each shoe on for me and fastened them as if I were a child. "Stand up," she commanded. I did. She pulled the shorts on over my bum and straightened the elastic at the waist. I grabbed my gym bag and my cane. Her friends looked uncomfortable. I thanked her, cringing at myself for doing so.

Even while it was happening, I wanted to respond differently, to tell her to stop. But I froze, stunned into silent compliance by her behavior. Somehow in her treatment of me, I lost my agency.

While the words and actions of the cabbie and the woman at the community center are notably harsh and dehumanizing, they reflect sentiments and behavior that are rife within our society.

Depictions of persons with disabilities in the media or literature or other arts reinforce stereotypes that promote objectification and prejudice. Rarely is a person with a disability presented as a multidimensional, complex character, driven by human desire, who just happens to possess physical challenges. Instead, they are lauded as inspirational heroes, victims, villains, or objects of pity. A few years ago, a British reality TV show that followed people with disabilities on dates chose the title *The Undateables.*

More than two decades of being disabled have affirmed for me that the social stigma and discrimination that people with disabilities face further extends to the ever-present struggle for access to services and built environments.

As a disabled person, I have learned that going out into the world is fraught with complications. Information on accessibility for restaurants, events, venues, offices, and buildings is inconsistently provided, and when it is, rarely do the words "barrier-free" appear. Listed under "accessibility" is often the number of stairs at the entrance and the flights required to access washrooms. And, since stairs render an establishment inaccessible, this information tells people with mobility disabilities that they're not welcome.

I do sometimes attend events in inaccessible locations. Once, I was helped up the stairs to a friend's birthday party, only to slide down again on my bum in full view of other guests, patrons, and staff at the end of the night. Could my friend have picked a more accessible space? Possibly, but they're in short supply.

Universal design, emphasizing the creation of environments that can be understood and used by as many people as possible, regardless of ability, would help anyone with mobility limitations experience the built environment more fully. In addition, the presence of people with disabilities in public spaces could lessen the prejudices all too present in our society.

It might also preclude the need to categorize oneself as

disabled, or even the need to prove "disability" to gain access to services and built environments. Ability exists along a continuum, comprised of visible and invisible conditions. We should all remember that.

I once attended a conference where a speaker reminded the audience that "able-bodiedness" is a temporary state. Whether from birth, illness, injury, or aging, many of us will need accessible services and environments.

Frankly, we deserve better.

AFTERWORD

While this book is based on my experience, some names have been changed and composite characters created. As well, some details and timing of events have been altered.

ACKNOWLEDGMENTS

I would like to thank Second Story Press for giving such a welcome home to my book, in particular Gillian Rodgerson for her warm support and enthusiasm. I am grateful for the editorial expertise of Diane Young, and the fabulous cover designed by Natalie Olsen. Many thanks to the rest of the team: Margie Wolfe, Phuong Truong, Melissa Kaita, Jordan Ryder, Emma Rodgers, Bronte Germain, and Michaela Stephen.

Thanks to Helen Humphreys for her mentorship and support of this book at Sage Hill Writing Experience many years ago, for her continued friendship, and for bringing the ever exuberant and joyful Fig into my life.

I am especially grateful to my friends for their encouragement and support in my writing and my life. Thanks to Kim Luke, Mira Hudson, Caroline Shecter, Zoe Ricketts, Marco Reiter, Kirsteen MacLeod, Kirsten Pollard, and Nancy Jo Cullen.

For their insight and guidance on early versions of the

book, I would like to thank my former writing group: Anthony De Sa, the late Bernard Grzyb, Rekha Lakra, Sheila Murray, James Papoutsis, and Susan Shuter.

For Stillpoint retreats, I am grateful to Maureen Garvie, Lori Vos, and Rebecca Gowan, for their considered and careful reading and input on the book, their friendship, and unwavering support.

Thank you to Cynthia Holz for reading and giving feedback on an initial draft of the manuscript.

I am also grateful to Darryl Tracy, physiotherapist and friend, for providing expert guidance on the book, and for his enthusiasm and support for my writing.

To my family—Joyce Mockler, Kathryn Mockler, David Poolman, Brian Shuter, and the late Helen Jeffrey for their support and encouragement.

Thank you to the Ontario Arts Council and the Toronto Arts Council for financial assistance while working on this book.

I am grateful for residencies at the Vermont Studio Center and the Tyrone Guthrie Centre in which portions of this book were written.

ABOUT THE AUTHOR

SUSAN MOCKLER is a disabled writer living in Kingston, Ontario. Her stories and essays have been published in Canada and the US, including work in *Voices From the FOLD: A Festival Magazine, Flash Fiction Magazine, 2020 Editor's Choice Award Winner, THIS Magazine, Geist, Descant, Ars Medica*, and *Taddle Creek.*

Susan has attended writing residencies in Ireland, Spain, the US, and Canada. She has received grants from the Ontario Arts Council and the Toronto Arts Council to support her writing.

Fractured: a memoir is her first book.